Clemens Conrad

Repetitive Strain Injury:
Personal Story & Treatment Options

All the information in this book is based on my personal experience during a three-year battle with the injury, supplemented by advice from other sufferers, websites, doctors and books. Even if your symptoms are similar, the cause may be a totally different one! I am not a doctor; I am only a former sufferer, who has dealt with this topic intensively. This book is designed to provide helpful information on the subjects discussed. It is not meant to be used, nor should it be used, to diagnose or treat any medical condition. For diagnosis or treatment of any medical problem consult your own physician and discuss the content of this book with him/her. The publisher and author are not responsible for any specific health needs that may require medical supervision and are not liable for any damages or negative consequences from any treatment, action, application or preparation, to any person reading or following the information in this book. References are provided for informational purposes only and do not constitute endorsement of any websites or other sources. Readers should be aware that the websites listed in this book may change.

I dedicate this book to my family and many friends. A special thank you to my parents, Anna, Felicitas, Julia and Claire.

Contents

Preface

During my illness I have grappled with the issue of RSI extensively. I realized that this particular disease is hardly known either to the general public or to the medical world. For this reason I decided to write down my experiences; to help others and to spread the word in general.

For many of us it is commonplace to sit at the computer for several hours each day but hardly anyone thinks about possible consequences of those repetitive finger movements. Before I experienced the severe pain, I would not have thought about it either and I certainly would not have listened to any warnings from others.

During the years of my battle with RSI I have been exposed to many limitations and I have also seen a wide range of possible consequences which were experienced by fellow sufferers. I was in pain holding a simple cup and I was unable to open bottles on my own. I experienced pain when eating with a knife and fork. I could not work on the computer or even write by hand. If both hands are affected, the quality of life is very restricted and in extreme cases living on your own is no longer possible. If you already suffer from mild discomfort, I strongly advise you to address that issue before it becomes worse.

If your RSI is a result of several years of stressful repetitive movements, unfortunately there is no way to fix this from one day to another. In advanced cases, you should give yourself about six months to regenerate. Initially you have to reduce the repetitive strain as much as possible. You will need approximately 60-90 minutes daily to perform the exercises described in this book.

The healing path of RSI is very bumpy. You will have very good days, but also severe relapses. Always try to think positively. There is a way out of this injury! The most important thing is that you never give up and lose hope.

My story in a nutshell

In 2006 I first experienced severe pain in my forearms after working on the computer intensively. I was 20 years old at that time.

In 2007 I had been seen by many doctors, but no one had any idea. Mid-year I couldn't even hold a cup without pain. I spent time on the internet and read a couple of English books on the topic of RSI.

2008: My condition improved significantly after setting up an ergonomic workstation and working with a physical therapist. I started publishing my experiences in German at the website www.repetitive-strain-injury.de

In 2009 I was almost healed. However, I still had to perform stretches and take short breaks regularly. I published my story as a German book.

In 2010 I had rebuilt all my muscles and I was able to work again on the computer just as before.

2015: Thousands of people have visited my website and/or have bought my book in the past years. To overcome the language barrier I decided to translate everything into English and publish it for free at www.rsipain.com and as a book.

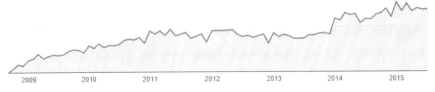

Why buy a book then?

- RSI sufferers usually do not want to spend much additional time on the computer.
- You can read it anywhere you like (even in the bath).
- You can easily mark certain passages.
- Speaking with a health professional is easier when bringing a real book rather than having to say "I have read (…) on the internet. What do you think?"

All information in this book is based on my personal experience during a three-year battle with the injury, supplemented by advice from other sufferers, websites, doctors and books. Even if your symptoms are similar, the cause may be a totally different one! I am not a doctor; I am only a former sufferer, who has dealt with this topic intensively. This book is designed to provide helpful information on the subjects discussed. It is not meant to be used, nor should it be used, to diagnose or treat any medical condition. For diagnosis or treatment of any medical problem consult your own physician and discuss the content of this book with him/her.

RSI Basics

What is RSI?

Definition

RSI is not a clearly defined medical term. Repetitive strain injury is an umbrella term for a variety of pain in muscles, tendons and nerves.[1] It primarily consists of micro-injuries of forearm tissue and includes diseases such as compression syndromes (nerve and blood vessels), tendinitis, tenosynovitis and myofascial trigger points.[2] However, an accurate diagnosis is difficult, because sufferers are often affected by more than one disease. On the other hand those micro-injuries cannot be detected with imaging techniques such as X-rays or MRI scans. In addition, the individual problems are often not very pronounced, but jointly cause the pain. In addition, long-term pain alters nerve cells so that after some time they already send out pain signals at low stresses and strains. If you visit a doctor after some time, you might still feel the pain, even if you had quit the repetitive movement which triggered the pain in the first place.

Causes

RSI is usually caused by repetitive movements performed over a longer period of time. Affected are office workers and PC/video game players (repetitive finger movements), assembly line workers (repetitive hand movements), cashiers (moving thousands of goods in the same direction every day), musicians, sign-language interpreters (up to 5600 movements per hour) etc. This list could go on and on, because in almost every profession there are monotonous tasks prevalent. The diseases mentioned above are not the actual causes, they are only a result of an unfavorable working posture and thousands of repeated movements.

Apart from purely physical reasons, there might also be psychological reasons for the pain *(see Causes, page 6).*

(Incorrect) Synonyms

Apart from "repetitive strain injury" there are various other terms used to describe those types of injuries: repetitive stress injury, CTD (cumulative trauma disorder) or OOS (occupational overuse syndrome), mouse arm, tennis

---

1 cf. Pascarelli, Emil; Quilter, Deborah (1994). Repetitive Strain Injury: A Computer User's Guide. New York: Wiley
2 cf. Peddie, Sandra; Rosenberg, Craig H (1999). The Repetitive Strain Injury Sourcebook. Los Angeles: Lowell House

and golfer's elbow, tendinitis, carpal tunnel syndrome. Mouse arm for example is a little misleading, because it suggests that the arm pain is solely caused by the mouse use. The keyboard plays an equally large part, if not even significantly more. As you can read in my *injury history (page 12)*, I was affected on both arms, although I operated the mouse just with my right hand.

Tennis and golfer's elbow are also sometimes used as a synonym for RSI, but really are just labels for a local irritation or inflammation of the elbow. Computer work can also cause a tennis elbow, but the tendon at the elbow is then usually just one of several pain spots. The relatively simple stretch for treating tennis and golfer's elbows is included in the far more extensive "RSI package". If you regularly play tennis, golf or a similar type of sport or perform technical work with your hands, respond to the special test *(see Tennis elbow, page 71)* and just rarely use a PC, then just focus on the corresponding stretching exercises.

Prevalence

RSI definitely is not a small issue. The "Occupational Safety and Health Administration" (OSHA) (which is an agency of the United States Department of Labor) already stated in 1996: "One in every three workers' compensation dollars pays for RSIs. In all, insurers awarded an estimated 2.73 million workers' compensation claims for RSIs in 1993, costing employers more than $20 billion. Indirect costs to employers are estimated to be five times that amount -- $100 billion. One major insurance company estimated the individual cost per claim to be $8,000, or double the average claim for other injuries or illnesses."[1]

Type of pain

Sufferers mostly complain about various pains in varying strength:

* Stabbing pain
* Diffuse pain
* Numbness
* Sensory disturbances
* Tingling
* Power loss
* Coldness
* Swelling

---

1 http://www.osha.gov/pls/oshaweb/owadisp.show_document?p_table=SPEECHES&p_id=206

Place of pain

RSI almost always manifests itself at several points on the upper body, in particular:

- Hands
- Wrists
- Forearms
- Elbows
- Shoulders
- Neck
- Back

Causes

In most cases Repetitive Strain Injury is caused by physical overload, but it can also have a psychological background. Currently known are the following primary causes:

1) Physical overload caused by repetitive motion
2) Psychosomatic causes
    a) Tension Myositis Syndrome
    b) Fear of RSI

The first time pain often occurs in very stressful situations. However, this stress is often only the trigger, not the cause. The longer the symptoms persist, the more psychological aspects play a role: fear of the future, fear of having to quit your current work, fear of never returning to a 100% healthy state. It does not matter if the primary cause is physical or psychological, after a few painful months these fears play a significant role.

Both causes result in **limited blood flow** whether due to tense and overstretched muscles (physical cause) or directly controlled by the central nervous system (psychosomatic cause). The reduced blood flow means an **insufficient supply of oxygen** and a **lack of removal of waste products**.

There are some forms of RSI that can be operated on. These are, for example, the ulnar nerve entrapment and carpal tunnel syndrome. These nerve compression symptoms may trigger the pain, but with computer users they are usually not the culprit. In particular the carpal tunnel syndrome (CTS) is too quickly diagnosed by some doctors. This is understandable, because surgery is possible and an apparent solution is found. But even in cases where the CTS diagnosis is correct and surgical intervention brings short-term relief, the pain often comes back after some time because the underlying causes (poor posture, stress, etc.) have not been addressed. If your doctor recommends surgery, you should obtain a second opinion. You should have exhausted all non-invasive options before being operated upon.

In the following section you will find more information about those three primary causes. I have created a diagram for each part illustrating a possible injury progression. Of course the scaling of the x-axis (January to December) is different for each person. In my case I would have to more than double the length, however most fellow sufferers have to halve the length. If your pain occurred only temporarily so far, it might already vanish by next week. The three causes do not always occur on an isolated basis, they can be mixed.

The straight progression of the line of the overall pain is a little misleading: A continuous improvement should occur over time, however it probably will not be that straightforward. It may happen that you feel really bad on one day and painless the next day. In general it can be said (which was confirmed to me by fellow sufferers) that initially the pain-free intervals become longer and the pain intensity subsides only slowly over time.

1) Physical overload

As described in the chapter *What is RSI? (page 3)*, a repetitive motion is the leading cause of RSI. Minimal tissue damage is usually repaired during rest periods (e.g. overnight). But if those rest periods are too short or the strain is too high, those small tissue damages add up until eventually a level is reached where your forearms start to ache.

"But I'm only moving my fingers, that's not exhausting?!" Well, it is. Thousands of repetitions do affect muscles, tendons, nerves and joints, even if the pain only becomes apparent after some time.

During a regular working day emails, reports, notes, etc. add up quickly to the amount of roughly four written A4 pages. With an average of 3,800 characters per page you move your fingers about 15,200 times. If you also consider text corrections and mouse clicks, a number of 20,000 adds up easily. Including private computer use in the evening, you have moved your fingers 25,000 times on a single day.

Compare that with a marathon: it takes about 50,000 steps. Do you think that it is healthy to run a half-marathon every day? And not just for a few weeks, but years or even decades? The long-term wear is obvious.

The load is distributed on more than two fingers when working on the computer, but the relatively small muscles in the forearm are also much less durable than leg muscles. In addition, office work usually takes place in an absolutely non-ergonomic position, so that the lack of oxygen supply is another negative factor.

In my case the years of extreme strain were also the cause of my pain. This most commonly encountered form of repetitive strain injury is also discussed extensively in this book.

Usually the first pain occurs after long, stressful work phases. If these warning signs are ignored for weeks, then the pain intensifies, occurs regularly and is often noticeable well into the evening. If you then still do not change your working attitude, posture and take regular breaks, the pain can become chronic and will not disappear completely even after longer periods of rest (e.g. vacation). The longer you ignore the pain and take no action, the more protracted will the recovery process become.

In the diagram you can see that the physical strain can be continuously reduced with frequent breaks, stretching etc. However, if you have ignored the first warning signs over a longer period (e.g. temporary mild pain in the wrist), then the healing might already take several months. The longer you feel the pain, the more you will doubt the healing ability of your body (which unquestionably exists!). Due to that fact, all sufferers should also have a look at the special chapter *Psyche (page 59)*.

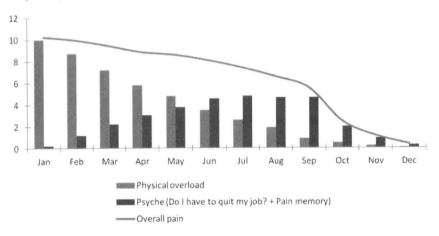

A frequent question is: "Why weren't these problems as widespread in the past (in the age of typewriters)?" The reasons are simple: lower typing speed, forced breaks when changing pages and after pressing the carriage return button and of course, there were much less people engaged in typing back then. Today there is almost no profession without office work.

2a) Psyche (Tension Myositis Syndrome)

RSI is not always a consequence of mere physical overload. As explained in the previous section, in most cases the psyche also plays a role (albeit minor). However, it can also be the main cause for some people! Some sufferers would normally stop reading now: "My pain is real, I am not imagining it!" Of course, your pain is real, but it may not be based on small tissue damage. The brain has the possibility to control the blood flow (and hence the supply of oxygen), so the pain might arise in some parts of the body. With this pain the brain tries to distract you from bad experiences / feelings or stress in the subconscious mind. Some examples are death of a family member / friend, divorce, problems with work colleagues / friends, illness of a family member / friend, new boss, debt. But also really positive changes in life can **subconsciously** trigger severe stress: moving, marriage, birth of a child etc.

Dr. John Sarno has researched this phenomenon for several decades and has given it the name Tension Myositis Syndrome (TMS). It might not only be the cause of pain in the arm, but can also affect the entire body. Among professionals, particularly traditional doctors and orthopedics, this theory is very controversial. However, in his book *The Mindbody Prescription*[1] Dr. Sarno refers to his high success rate of several thousand patients and various success stories confirm his theory.

"How do I know that I am affected by TMS?" This question is not easy to answer because the stress is subconscious and not always easy to pinpoint. If you work on the computer (or do comparable RSI-risk activities) for significantly less than half of your working hours or you only recently started to work intensively on the computer (1-2 years), then you should consider TMS as a possible cause for your pain. Even if you do not believe that you are affected by TMS you should check out the information in the chapter *Psyche (page 59)* (other complaints such as back pain or headaches and even depression can be also triggered by TMS).

In the next diagram you can see that with a "classic" Tension Myositis Syndrome the physical overload only plays a subordinate role. In addition, the longer you do not address your suppressed emotions, the more likely it is that you develop fears of the future.

---

1 Sarno, John E. (1999). The Mindbody Prescription: Healing the Body, Healing the Pain. New York: Warner Books

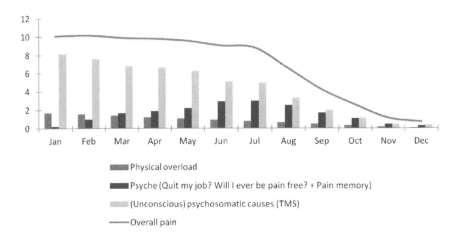

Physical overload

Psyche (Quit my job? Will I ever be pain free? + Pain memory)

(Unconscious) psychosomatic causes (TMS)

Overall pain

2b) Psyche (fear of RSI)

A colleague has been on sick leave with severe pain in both forearms for several weeks? Your company gives a training session on "healthy working" and you realize that you have had poor posture for the last couple of years? You work six hours a day or more on the PC? You have read my medical history? You work overtime to finish an important project?

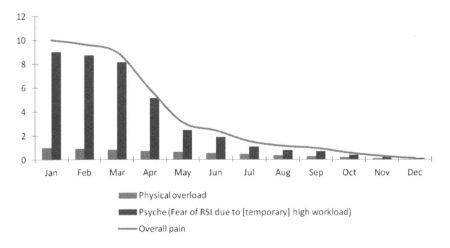

Physical overload

Psyche (Fear of RSI due to [temporary] high workload)

Overall pain

The mere fear of RSI can paradoxically trigger RSI. If you think about the possible dire consequences of your work all the time, you almost automatically tense up and won't move naturally. As a result the blood flow deteriorates and you feel pain - a self-fulfilling prophecy.

Have a look at the appropriate section in the chapter *Psyche (page 59)*, no one needs to develop repetitive strain injury!

My Story

History

I felt pain for the first time in July 2006, and I was just 20 years old. Not necessarily an age at which you would expect something like this to happen. During the nineties private households became much more "technical": computers, game consoles and cell phones, all increased the strain on our hands and fingers significantly. Meanwhile, I have experienced how painful these thousand-fold repetitions of muscles, tendons, joints and nerves can be.

Starting with Tetris on the Game Boy, I quickly switched to computer games: flight simulators, auto racing, strategy games and first person shooters. The Internet came over the analog phone line at snail's pace (if at all) and was expensive compared to today's prices. Wikipedia and Google did not exist, homework was still written by hand and cell phones were not common.

I want to clarify the fact that my hand strain from the age of 7 to 14 was still moderate (compared to today's children).

As a teenager I initially played intensely on the computer (often several hours a day). As time went by I discovered my enthusiasm for creating websites, so I predominantly switched to that kind of work in my free time. Furthermore I coded some software in computer science class and at home. At the weekends I worked at a local computer store. All my internships I completed involved computers in some form. Even in the 9 months of my community service (compulsory in Germany at that time) I was able to contribute my computer skills. I also started a small business for PC services and web design.

Up to this point I never felt pain in my hands or forearms after working on the computer. I had not thought about taking short breaks in between to give the body time to recover. If someone had made me aware of this risk, I probably would not have listened. I would not have been able to imagine the tremendous pain that could occur.

My hand strain from the age of 14 to 20 was above average at that time.

With the constant advance in technology in all areas of life, the average strain on our hands will increase significantly in the coming years and decades. Consequently my prediction is that hand-forearm discomfort due to repetitive strain (=repetitive strain injuries) will increase in the future. As a cure is much more difficult than prevention, I would like to be actively involved with this book to help avoid that kind of pain. Abstract warnings will probably fall on deaf ears with 99% of all people (I would not have reacted differently). Only those who already feel pain themselves will deal with this issue and take the risk seriously.

I hope to reach a few doubters with this personal story. Even though I might only convince a handful of people to listen to their body and treat it well, my work on this book will already have paid off!

The rest of this chapter deals with the chronological course of my injury. I don't mention all diagnoses and treatments, I limit myself to the most significant. Text passages in *italic* are retrospective comments.

July 2006

At the end of a three-month internship I felt a slight pain in my right wrist for the first time. In the following days I continued to work normally, hoping that after the next weekend everything would be okay again - but it was not. Even switching the mouse to my left hand did not help significantly. The pain had intensified within a week and now both wrists were already equally affected. At the weekend both forearms swelled so much that the armband of my wristwatch was too short to wear it any more. My doctor diagnosed a tendon irritation and prescribed me diclofenac gel and ibuprofen 400 tablets. His prognosis: In one to two weeks everything should be back to normal.

RSI often does not develop that fast. Usually there are warning signs in advance in the form of temporary, mild discomfort.

August 2006

After three weeks with tablets and gels the swelling had gone, the severe pain in both forearms remained (even with no workload). The former tendon irritation was now labeled tenosynovitis by my doctor. Cortisone injections in both elbows only brought relief for the same day.

I don't recommend cortisone treatments because long-term tissue damage is a risk and the positive effect on me was minimal.

September 2006

Since the beginning of the pain I had hardly worked on the PC. Any additional activity using my hands was greatly reduced as well. This absolute rest had a significant negative effect on my physical fitness. Deep friction massages reduced the pain at times of rest. I had to stop weight training (as prescribed by a physical therapist) because of significant pain after the first exercises.

Strengthening exercises could have helped me, but only at a much later stage. If you still feel constant pain during rest, you shouldn't do strengthening exercises. Instead I should have gone out for a jog more often.

October - December 2006

In October I enrolled in university (business informatics). The pain had become less after wearing wrist braces and resting for the last two and a half months. I was still far from being pain free, but at least I was able to do some work on the PC.

The second orthopedist I consulted did not know anything more to help me but to send me to a natural health professional. She diagnosed a heavy metal poisoning and ordered a detoxification.

In addition to the stabbing pain I now felt slight sensory disturbances. Especially when the arms were poorly supplied with blood, I felt a strange feeling in both forearms. I had never experienced this feeling before. It was diffusely affecting the entire forearm: no real pain, but as a constant feeling it was very uncomfortable.

The detoxification was a waste of time and money (later performed hair and blood tests were negative). In addition I didn't inform myself further about the condition called "RSI" which I read about on the Internet.

January - March 2007

Both osteopath and chiropractor agreed that my arm pain originated from my spine. They carried out several spinal adjustments which always brought short-term improvements. I was also given a quick introduction into trigger point massage which proved to be helpful as well. They informed me about the importance of an ergonomic posture and showed me core strengthening exercises. My neck and back pain completely vanished. My main problem however, the severe pain during activities involving the hands (e.g. PC work or handwriting texts), did not improve.

In retrospect I cannot understand why no doctor showed interest in my hints about working intensively with computers. Instead heavy metal poisoning, too tightly curved cervical vertebrae, a minor bicycle accident or past sports injuries were pinpointed as probable cause. Why did no one see that the strain I was under doing office work simply was too much for my body to absorb? Apparently very few doctors in Germany know this condition, although RSI affects so many people.

April - June 2007

The discomfort in my left arm improved slightly, but not in my right arm. My muscles were weak. The one year long rest took its toll, my muscles cramped after just a couple of minutes working. I had largely abandoned note-taking in lectures. Instead I had to photocopy the notes of fellow students.

In addition to the pain sensory disturbances sporadically occurred (I could not see a link between office work and those sensory disturbances).

A doctor specialized in Traditional Chinese Medicine (TCM) was very surprised that none of the previous doctors had recommended stretching exercises for my forearms.

Since I wore wrist braces most of the time, my wrist mobility was greatly diminished. The stretching exercises he recommended were absolutely right, but I should have started more gently.

July - September 2007

Regular massages and stretching exercises helped to soften my forearm muscles. I now had returned to my own RSI diagnosis and informed myself in detail about this condition on the Internet and with the book *It's Not Carpal Tunnel Syndrome! RSI Theory and Therapy for Computer Professionals*[1]. The renowned hand surgery department of a hospital hadn't heard of RSI and showed no interest to take a closer look at the issue. They only referred me to another orthopedist.

I visited an orthopedics department of another hospital and was met with much more patience and kindness. A senior physician knew the term RSI, saw my office work as the cause and after more than a year confirmed my own diagnosis!

October 2007 - January 2008

With gentle strengthening exercises I could stop the progressive loss of muscle mass. However the pain in my right forearm was still stronger than in my left forearm and overall I felt no improvement. The visits to a pain therapist and a psychologist brought no new information.

---

1 Damany, Suparna; Bellis, Jack (2000). It's Not Carpal Tunnel Syndrome! RSI Theory and Therapy for Computer Professionals. Philadelphia: Simax

February - July 2008

It was obvious that despite a correct diagnosis and appropriate exercises there was no improvement. As a consequence I quit university and reduced the PC work to give my body the proper time to recover.

Thanks to the advice of a former RSI sufferer I visited a Vojta therapist (also known as reflex locomotion). She helped me overcome my poor posture and we worked together on strengthening my muscles. Initially I saw her once a week, later every two weeks. I bought ergonomic equipment for my home office, performed stretching exercises, nerve mobilization, trigger point massages. I started doing a lot more sport activities, read everything I found about pain memory and other psychological factors. All that improved the blood flow and hence reduced my overall pain. Simultaneously I slowly increased the PC work and began creating a German website about my RSI story.

RSI is a very complex issue that is influenced by many factors. With the extent of this book you can easily see that it is not possible for a doctor to give you all the essential information about what to do in the average five to ten minutes consultation. What you should expect however, is a correct diagnosis and a recommendation to other resources (books, websites …). That would not only help the patient, but would also be in the interest of our expensive health system (at least from the point of view of a health insurance).

For me it was the right decision temporarily to stop working on a computer. Fortunately most RSI sufferers don't have to go that far because their pain is less severe and they can also start earlier with the proper countermeasures. Only if you are affected as long as I was, other diseases are ruled out and there is absolutely no improvement, you should think of the option I chose.

August - October 2008

Following the significant improvement in the summer, it was time to take up another university class. I chose a distance university this time to be able to take regular breaks and to divide my working time flexibly. I dismissed business informatics this time because I didn't want to push my luck and I chose business studies instead. With that degree I can still enter the IT sector later on if I want to.

November 2008 - July 2009

The last few months were very positive: pain at times of rest is almost completely gone. I can do pull-ups and push-ups again! Only after working on the computer for several hours my forearms remind me of the importance of short breaks. What I have noticed very clearly in this phase is that if you have not used your muscles for years it takes the same amount of time to fully regenerate. And as long as the muscles have not regained their original strength, we should not expect to be able to work long hours.

August 2009 - July 2010

For the past year I have been working on the computer for many hours a day. Pain at times of rest only occurred after I overdid things. My muscle strength is also back to normal. If you do not feel any pain, you easily slip back into poor posture and bad working habits.

August 2010 - September 2015

There hasn't been any significant pain since the last entry. After an entire day working on the PC my forearms feel a bit "different", but that could be due to my increased awareness of the issue. It doesn't restrict me at all.

Medical diagnoses

During my illness I have visited several primary care physicians, orthopedists, osteopaths, a chiropractor, two neurologists, a sports physical therapist, two physical therapists, a masseuse, a homeopath, the hand surgery of a renowned hospital, the orthopedics department of another hospital, a pain therapist and a psychologist.

With two exceptions, no one knew the term RSI. Even worse, **several times I was told that pain due to excessive computer use cannot occur!** At the same time they found several (alleged) other problems. The diagnoses from some doctors were correct, but described only parts of my problem. Incidentally, there was no difference between private and public medical care.

Diagnoses in chronological order (same diagnoses from different doctors are listed just once):

- Tendon irritation
- Tenosynovitis
- Tennis elbow
- Heavy metal poisoning
- Thoracic and cervical spine blockages
- Irritated nerves in the forearm
- Tilting the head results in "deactivating" some arm muscles
- Pronation of the cervical spine
- Lumbar fixation; cervical spondylosis; shoulder-arm syndrome, myogelosis, myalgia
- Paresthesias in both arms
- Unclear wrist symptoms on both sides
- Too tightly curved cervical vertebrae
- Persistent epicondylitis radialis combined with myofascial pain, muscular imbalance, nerve root compression ruled out, cervical spine dysfunction C5/6
- Chronic wrist instability
- Various shortened muscles
- Muscle trigger points in the region of both forearms and finger extensors (in accord with Travell and Simons)

- Significant, autonomic dysregulation with excessive skin reaction to pressure and touch (redness) and very pale hands, looking like a glove

Treatment / medication

Almost every doctor had a different idea to solve my problem. The following table is a chronological list of what I have done; with the respective failure/success. Duplicate treatments are listed just once.

Treatment / medication	Impact felt
Initially avoided any activity with the hands	The pain didn't become worse
Diclofenac gel for my forearms and ibuprofen 400 tablets for three weeks	The swelling of my forearms decreased after three weeks
X-ray of wrist and elbow	No abnormalities identifiable
3x cortisone injections in both elbows	Pain-free for one day
Epicondylitis clasps for both arms	None
Weeks of absolute rest (very little movement)	Slight improvement
Neurological examination of the forearms	No abnormalities identifiable
11x deep friction massages	Less pain at times of rest
Strengthening exercises in a gym	Significant deterioration, aborted
8x electrical muscle stimulation (forearms)	Only short-term improvement
Wore wrist braces constantly for two weeks	Slight improvement
Six weeks spirulina maxima algae tablets and essence of cilantro	None
Hair and blood analysis (suspected heavy metal poisoning)	Suspicion could not be confirmed
Food supplements (yeast, selenium, zinc, vitamin C)	None
Running	Temporarily completely free of symptoms (as with any other activity which increased blood flow to the forearms)

For acute symptoms: cold water (or hot-cold contrast baths)	Short-term relief
Spinal adjustments, osteopathic treatments	Slight (temporary) improvement
Massaging various trigger points	Slight improvement
MRI of the cervical spine	Tightly curved cervical vertebrae, but no other abnormalities identified
Standing upright, stretching neck muscles	Less neck pain
Exercises to stabilize the back area, sitting ball in my home office	No more back and neck pain
Neck and back massage	Slight improvement
Stretching exercises for both arms	Increased the pain in my wrists, therefore abandoned after two days
Blood test (arthritis, rheumatism)	No abnormalities
MRI of the right wrist with contrast agent	No abnormalities
Piroxicam 20mg tablets	Less pain
PH-examination of my blood	Rather sour, but still within the tolerance range
Ergonomic working posture, ergonomic equipment, regular breaks, stretching, strengthening, nerve mobilization, stimulating blood flow and massaging of specific trigger points (supported by a physical therapist)	**Slow, but steady recovery**
Erase pain memory	**Final improvement**

The strengthening exercises I performed in a gym were started too early. They could have been helpful, but my muscles were already too weak. Furthermore, I initially did the stretching exercises too intensely.

Some other treatments were also helpful. But since there was no "master plan" and no one told me that the treatment could take half a year or longer (the most common information was 2-3 weeks), I stopped the massages, stretching etc. too early. I was also very confused from contradictory recommendations (complete rest <=> stretching exercises).

The website of Justin Bennett[1] and the book *It's Not Carpal Tunnel Syndrome!: RSI Theory and Therapy for Computer Professionals*[2] gave me hope that I'm on the right track. Those two sources of information were the reason why I created this book: to provide fellow sufferers with sensible tips for the prevention and treatment of RSI.

The exercises described in this book are usually sufficient for the prevention and cure of mild cases of RSI. If you are in a stage of chronic pain you should definitely consult an appropriate health professional. Ideally, he or she has already successfully treated other RSI patients.

---

1 http://www.howibeatrsi.com
2 Damany, Suparna; Bellis, Jack (2000). It's Not Carpal Tunnel Syndrome! RSI Theory and Therapy for Computer Professionals. Philadelphia: Simax

What you can do

Prevention (summary)

Office employees suffer from daily strains while doing repetitive actions (typing and using the mouse). Combined with bad sitting posture these "small" strains can already lead to pain, reduced sensation or even numbness in fingers, wrists, arms and shoulders as well as in the neck area after some years of high workload.

This problem (known as Repetitive Strain Injury, RSI) is avoidable in most cases if you adapt an ergonomic posture and take regular micro breaks.

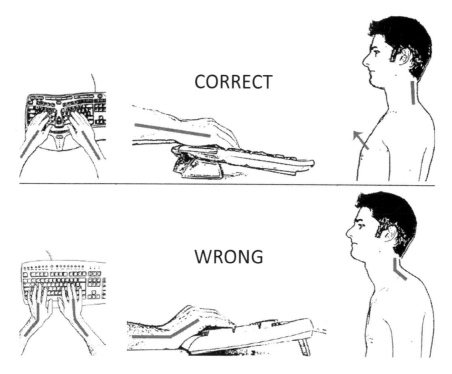

Sit actively

Do not remain in the same position for several hours, keep your body moving. If you are not currently using the keyboard or mouse, rest your hands in your lap.

23

Take regular breaks

Instead of having a few long breaks, take shorter breaks more often (shake out your hands and arms at least every five minutes, stand up every half an hour). Look out of the window at a distant object regularly to relax your eyes.

Keep your elbows close to your waist

The distance between your body and the keyboard should be minimal so that you do not have to reach out with your hands while typing. Keep your elbows close to your waist and the mouse next to the keyboard.

Use ergonomic equipment

Select from the wide range of ergonomic mice and keyboards. If possible, work on a height-adjustable desk and regularly use speech recognition software.

Treatment plans

The RSI treatment that helps everyone affected best does not exist. RSI is too complex, there are different causes and consequences. The severity and duration of the pain can vary enormously.

I have divided the healing process into five phases and created corresponding treatment plans, so each sufferer can pick the most suitable exercises. No matter which stage you have reached, you should consult a doctor and discuss the measures proposed in this book with him.

Phase	Duration of pain	Pain intensity	Swelling of the forearms
First phase	Permanently	Very strong	Yes
Second phase	Regularly to permanently	Strong	None or slight
Third phase	Regularly	Medium to strong	-
Fourth phase	Sporadically to regularly	Low to medium	-
Fifth phase	-	-	-

This book is designed to provide helpful information on the subjects discussed. It is not meant to be used, nor should it be used, to diagnose or treat any medical condition. For diagnosis or treatment of any medical problem consult your own physician and discuss the content of this book with him/her.

Treatment \ Phase	1	2	3	4	5 Prevention
Ergonomic workplace *(p. 29)*	X	X	X	X	X
Work habits *(p. 37)* + Work attitude *(p. 62)*	X	X	X	X	X
Read other personal stories[1]	X	X	X	X	
Pain diary *(p. 70)*	X	X	X	X	
Treat swelling *(p. 69)*	X				
Minimize workload	X	X			
Reduce workload			X	X	
Erase pain memory *(p. 66)*			X	X	
Stimulate blood flow *(p. 68)*		X	X	X	X
Relaxation techniques *(p. 69)*		X	X	X	X
Deep friction massage *(p. 75)*			X		
Stretching (active *p. 43* + passive *p. 48*)		X	X	X	X
Trigger point massage *(p. 49)*		X	X	X	X
Nerve mobilization *(p. 52)*			X	X	X
Strengthening *(p. 54)*				X	X

The following treatment plans only list exercises and activities that are not general in nature (e.g. ergonomic workstation, proper work habits).

1 http://www.rsipain.com/other-personal-stories.php

First phase

If your pain is very strong and you are in the first phase, you should as a first step minimize the strain on the affected body part (often the right forearm). Before proceeding to the exercises of the second phase, an existing swelling should be almost completely subsided *(page 69)*.

Second phase

Monday	Tuesday	Wednesday	Thursday	Friday	Saturday	Sunday
	Running (at least 30 minutes)			Running (at least 30 minutes)		Running (at least 30 minutes)
Stretching	Stretching	Stretching	Stretching	Stretching	Stretching	Stretching
Trigger point massage		Trigger point massage			Trigger point massage	
Stretching	Stretching	Stretching	Stretching	Stretching	Stretching	Stretching
Relaxation techniques	Relaxation techniques	Relaxation techniques	Relaxation techniques	Relaxation techniques	Relaxation techniques	Relaxation techniques

Third phase

Monday	Tuesday	Wednesday	Thursday	Friday	Saturday	Sunday
	Running (at least 30 minutes)			Running (at least 30 minutes)		Swimming
Stretching	Stretching	Stretching	Stretching	Stretching	Stretching	Stretching
Trigger point massage	Nerve mobilization	Trigger point massage	Nerve mobilization		Trigger point massage	Nerve mobilization
	Deep friction massage			Deep friction massage		
Stretching	Stretching	Stretching	Stretching	Stretching	Stretching	Stretching
Erase pain memory	Erase pain memory	Erase pain memory	Erase pain memory	Erase pain memory	Erase pain memory	Erase pain memory
Relaxation techniques	Relaxation techniques	Relaxation techniques	Relaxation techniques	Relaxation techniques	Relaxation techniques	Relaxation techniques

Fourth phase

Monday	Tuesday	Wednesday	Thursday	Friday	Saturday	Sunday
	Running (at least 30 minutes)			Running (at least 30 minutes)		Swimming
Stretching	Stretching	Stretching	Stretching	Stretching	Stretching	Stretching
Trigger point massage	Nerve mobilization	Trigger point massage	Nerve mobilization		Trigger point massage	Nerve mobilization
	Strengthe-ning			Strengthe-ning		
Stretching	Stretching	Stretching	Stretching	Stretching	Stretching	Stretching
Erase pain memory	Erase pain memory	Erase pain memory	Erase pain memory	Erase pain memory	Erase pain memory	Erase pain memory
Relaxation techniques	Relaxation techniques	Relaxation techniques	Relaxation techniques	Relaxation techniques	Relaxation techniques	Relaxation techniques

Fifth phase

Monday	Tuesday	Wednesday	Thursday	Friday	Saturday	Sunday
	Running (at least 30 minutes)			Running (at least 30 minutes)		Swimming
Trigger point massage			Nerve mobilization			
	Strengthe-ning			Strengthe-ning		
Stretching	Stretching	Stretching	Stretching	Stretching	Stretching	Stretching
Relaxation techniques	Relaxation techniques	Relaxation techniques	Relaxation techniques	Relaxation techniques	Relaxation techniques	Relaxation techniques

Note for TMS-Sufferers

If the cause of your RSI is psychological, then you can largely do without all the advice in this chapter. But a few stretches won't hurt and might protect you from possible future physical strain.

Equipment

An ergonomic workplace with the proper equipment is essential for healthy, sustainable office activity. In this chapter you will find the most important aspects with specific product recommendations. **The life cycle of technical products is quite short, so you should have a look at the corresponding page on my website**[1]. I constantly try to test new ergonomic products and will update or replace recommendations.

Monitor brightness

To prevent eyestrain, the contrast between the monitor and the surrounding area should be as small as possible. If your workplace is not optimally illuminated, you should lower the brightness of your monitor.

Monitor distance

The optimum viewing distance to the monitor is about an arm's length. If you sit too far away, it may happen that you let your head slip forward. The screen should be placed right in front of you so that you don't have to turn your head or upper body.

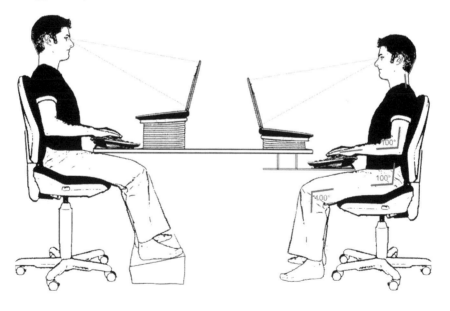

---

1 http://www.rsipain.com/equipment.php

Monitor height

The top edge of your monitor should be placed a few centimeters below eye level, so you can look down slightly while working.

If you work on a laptop you can use the corresponding docking station (if available), a universal laptop stand or you could increase the height with some magazines.

Desk

The standard height of a desk suits normal activities, however it is a bit too high when working with a keyboard. The best option is a height-adjustable desk that you can adjust according to your height and current activity. From time to time you can use it as a standing desk as well, so that you don't have to sit all day. An alternative is a regular desk with a lower-lying keyboard tray (see image, right person). When using the keyboard, elbow, hip and knee should have an angle of about 100°.

If you work on a standard desk and are not exceptionally large, either your feet dangle in the air or your elbow angle is less than 100° (which would be restricting blood flow). You can get by with a foot rest (see image, left person).

You should arrange your workplace in a way that your desk stands parallel to the window. That way you avoid a high contrast between the monitor and the bright background outside and you don't have sun reflections on the screen.

Standing desk

Working at a regular desk all day can cause stress on your back. A better option would be a height-adjustable desk (see above) which is relatively expensive though. A cheaper alternative is a bar table, combined with a large wooden plate from the DIY market and a block of wood for tilting the working surface (with a glued rubber lip, so that the 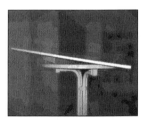 wooden plate does not slip out of position). Such a standing desk can be easily used for all private desk work at home.

Office chair

A good office chair is height-adjustable, has proper lumbar support, a tiltable backrest and seating surface and the backrest angle can be fixed or remain variable. The variable setting supports "active sitting", which means that you are constantly moving your body. A professional chair lets you adjust the pressure of the backrest to the individual weight of the user. Armrests are recommended, but only if they are height-adjustable and relatively short (so that you can work closely to your desk) and can be adjusted to your shoulder width. An office chair should be tested and bought in a specialty store. There you also get expert advice on the correct settings.

Seat cushion

A balance disc is an air-filled disc, which can be placed onto any chair. It serves the same purpose as a sitting ball, it stimulates a moving body, thus preventing tension in the back, shoulder and neck area. At the same time, it doesn't have the disadvantages of a sitting ball (no back support, risk of accident) and is portable at the same time. I recommend alternating between using the office chair with and without a balance disc.

Book stand / document holder

Newspapers, magazines, books, documents, etc. usually lie on a desk while reading. You have to tilt your head forward which strains your neck muscles. Give them a rest with the help of a book stand.

Ergonomic keyboard

An ergonomic keyboard should ideally meet the following three criteria:

1. A split key field to avoid bending your wrists to the outside (your tendons would irritate their tendon sheaths).

2. A palm rest to avoid bending your wrists to the upside (your tendons would irritate their tendon sheaths). Even better would be a keyboard with a negative tilt (backwards).

3. A curved key field (higher in the central section) to reduce the twisting of your forearms (you relieve your muscles and support the blood flow).

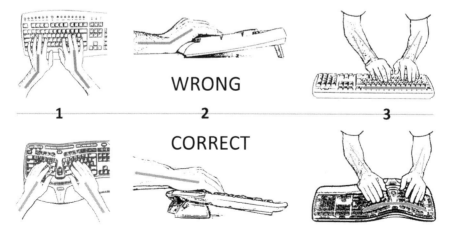

31

Recommendation:

Microsoft Natural Ergonomic Keyboard 4000: The Natural Ergonomic Keyboard 4000 prevents bending of the wrists and reduces the twisting of the forearms. I have been using this as my main keyboard for a couple of years now with great satisfaction. It is a bit too wide for right-handers however. Due to the number pad your right mouse arm is located a bit too far away from your body. That's one of the reasons why I switched to using the mouse with my left hand. There is an optional front riser to achieve a negative tilt (and I gladly use it). Overall the keyboard is a bit too high. That could have been engineered better. Despite everything it still is my favorite keyboard.

If the purchase of a new keyboard is not possible, you should use an additional wrist rest with your existing keyboard. That at least avoids bending your wrists to the upside.

If you suffer from shoulder and neck pain rather than from forearm pain, then a fourth aspect is important: the <u>width of the keyboard</u>. The number pad broadens the keyboard and the mouse use puts strain on your right shoulder/back area.

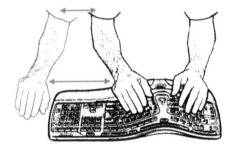 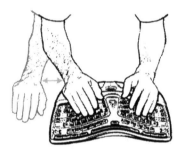

Possibilities with shoulder and neck pain:

1. <u>Narrow keyboard</u> without a number pad (e.g. *Microsoft Sculpt Ergonomic Keyboard*)
2. <u>Mouse in front of the keyboard</u> (see recommendations in this chapter)
3. <u>Left hand usage</u> (you will need one or two weeks to get used to this switch)

Ergonomic Mouse

With a conventional mouse your forearm lies flat on the table and the wrist is bent upwards (top right image). With each mouse click the tendon of your index finger irritates its tendon sheath. Instead, the wrist should be as straight as possible. You can either use a wrist rest or a special mouse. The wrist rest has the disadvantages that it promotes wrist movements (rather than larger arm movements) which might aggravate existing wrist pain and it could negatively affect blood flow.

Thus I prefer ergonomic mice which also allow straight wrists and reduce forearm twisting (ulna and radius are almost parallel, left image). You will need about two weeks to be able to work as effective as before.

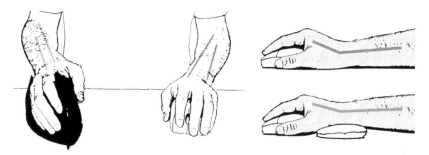

Depending on the type and location of your pain, different mice may be useful. The selection of your favorite mouse is a very individual decision. Even people with similar pain often assess the same model very differently.

If you primarily feel pain in the **wrist and forearm** and little to none in the neck/shoulder area, your hand should be able to rest on the mouse while using it. The movements should come out of the entire arm.

Recommendations:

Hippus HandShoe Mouse: This mouse appears to be of excellent quality, it fits your hand comfortably and requires only a short adjustment period. It is offered in three different sizes (measure the distance from your wrist up to the tip of the ring finger: < 17cm [small] | 17-19cm [medium] | > 19cm [large]). Each size is available as a wired and wireless version. I particularly recommended this mouse for the prevention and if you only have minor pain.

E-Quill AirO2bic: I have been using the E-Quill-mouse for years and I really like it. The movements come out of the entire arm, even more so compared to the Hippus mouse. It is made of very cheap looking plastic, which does not match the price level. Nevertheless, I never had any problem with it and it still works as on day one. The slope of the hand support is very steep, but it fits my idea of a neutral forearm posture.

3M Ergonomic Mouse: The 3M Ergonomic Mouse looks like a joystick, but the "stick" is not movable. It was my first ergonomic mouse and helped me get rid of the pain in my right wrist. The thumb operates the two mouse buttons on the top. Especially if your index and/or middle finger cause pain while working with a regular mouse, this mouse could be a good alternative. I wouldn't recommend it for years-long use, because the increased thumb usage might create pain itself after some time (especially if you are sending a lot of text messages with your mobile). You shouldn't clutch it, but hold your hand relaxed. It is available in two different sizes.

If you primarily feel pain in the **shoulder area**, then a small keyboard is important so that you can use the mouse closely to your body. Secondly, you should use a (standard) mouse, where you bend the wrist (=your forearm rests on the table). Alternatively, you could also use a roller bar mouse directly in front of the keyboard or you could try a graphics tablet.

Recommendations:

Mousetrapper Advance: The Mousetrapper works similarly to a laptop touchpad. It is placed in front of the keyboard, so that you don't have to reach out with your mouse arm. The adjustment period is short (because of the similarity to laptop touchpad).

Rollermouse: The Rollermouse is very similar to the Mousetrapper. But instead of a touchpad you operate the cursor by moving a rotatable bar with your fingers. I like it as well and also the adjustment period is surprisingly short.

Wacom Intuos Pen and Touch: For people who often work with image editing programs, a graphics tablet is the perfect option. With the precision of accustomed finger/hand movements, you can be more productive than with a regular mouse. But even with regular PC work, I see advantages over a standard mouse. However, if you still write a lot with pen and paper, then you might opt for the Mousetrapper or Rollermouse instead, in order to have a bit more variety during the day. The Wacom Intuos Pen and Touch can be operated with finger movements or with the corresponding pen. It is available in different sizes.

If the pain is located in your **index or middle finger**, then a mouse with a thumb button might be the best option. In addition to that, you should use an auto click program.

Recommendation:

3M Ergonomic Mouse: The 3M Ergonomic Mouse looks like a joystick, but the "stick" is not movable. It was my first ergonomic mouse and helped me get rid of the pain in my right wrist. The thumb operates the two mouse buttons on the top. Especially if your index and/or middle finger cause pain while working with a regular mouse, this mouse could be a good alternative. I wouldn't recommend it for years-long use, because the increased thumb usage might create pain itself after some time (especially if you are sending a lot of text messages with your mobile). You shouldn't clutch it, but hold your hand relaxed. It is available in two different sizes.

However, even using an ergonomic mouse if you have a stiff body posture this is unhealthy if done several hours a day. As long as you do not have to move the mouse or press a mouse button, put your hands in your lap and relax. It is also important that you get up every now and then and shake out your arms. The use of two simultaneously connected mice (left and right) can spread the strain on both hands thus reducing the risk of injury. If you already are in chronic pain, use different hand postures and mouse surfaces to erase the pain memory *(page 66)*.

All recommended ergonomic mice appear to be expensive, at least compared to standard $5 models. But if an ergonomic mouse can prevent just one sick day due to pain, it has already paid for itself (financially for the employer and health wise for the employee). Since RSI doesn't usually subside after only one day (a sick leave for several weeks or even months is not uncommon), much money can be saved in the long run.

Speech Recognition Software

When writing texts on the PC voice recognition software is by far the greatest relief available. In my opinion, it brings a much greater relief than the best ergonomic keyboard could ever achieve. You speak into a microphone and the software writes down everything you say. In the past the recognition quality was not good. Nowadays you can already work productively after a very short training period.

Properties	Dragon NaturallySpeaking 13 Home	Dragon NaturallySpeaking 13 Premium	Windows 8.1 (speech recognition is included)
Languages	English	English	English, German, French, Spanish, Japanese, Chinese
Supported programs	Basic dictation works with any program. In addition, some programs are supported with special voice commands.		Most Microsoft programs are supported, many others unfortunately not.
Microphone included	Yes		No
Profile export	No	Yes	No
Supported operating systems	Windows 7, 8	Windows 7, 8	Windows 8

If you have a Mac you can use Dragon Dictate, the functionality is roughly equivalent to the Windows Premium version

For the first couple of months I worked with the built-in Windows speech recognition. Then I switched to Dragon, mainly because of the better support of non-Microsoft programs. Writing longer texts with Dragon is considerably more relaxed than typing on a keyboard, so I also recommend this software to people without wrist pain. People who aren't fast at typing also benefit from not having to worry about where the letters are located on the keyboard.

If you do not have an external microphone, I recommend a cheap, but perfectly adequate headset. If your laptop has no microphone input, you have to choose a USB headset.

An internal laptop microphone is not sufficient and will produce bad results.

I use many of the products presented here every day and they make my life so much better. But they don't just help RSI sufferers, they also help to prevent injuring yourself in the first place.

Work habits

The most important concept in this context is "variation". You can always sit non-ergonomically, relax in an armchair while surfing the net etc. That's no problem, as long as you do not behave like that all the time. Stay active and do not work in one stiff posture for several hours: Our bodies need the variation!

A good working posture at a non-ergonomic workplace is better than having ergonomic equipment with a bad working posture. Ideally, of course, combine the ergonomic equipment with a correct working posture.

Posture

Work posture

We automatically hold our head in a way that our eyes can easily look forward horizontally.

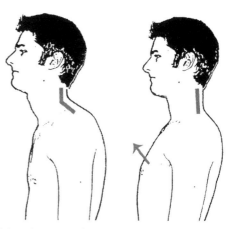

If you have a slack posture, you automatically move your head forward, which results in your upper back and neck being bent (see left image).

Imagine a string which pulls your chest upwards (right image, arrow). That will result in a straight neck and a natural spine.

The angle of the elbow joint should be about 100°. But again, as with many other recommendations: vary the execution.

Sit actively

Do not remain in the same position for several hours, move your upper body regularly. You can move your shoulders forward and backward in small circles, stretch your upper body in all directions and spread out your arms vertically above your head. Do that at least once every 30 minutes, the more - the better.

Keyboard-waist-distance

The gap between your upper body and the keyboard should be as small as possible, so that you don't have to stretch your arms forward and put strain on your shoulders. Make sure that your elbows are close to your body. A temporary working position could even be that you put the keyboard on your lap and use it there.

Don't bend your wrists while typing

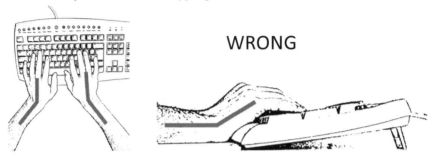

You should make sure that you don't bend your wrists while typing (ideally supported by an ergonomic keyboard).

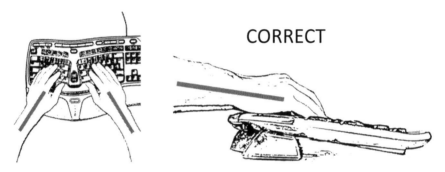

Use the mouse close to your body

If you are right-handed and use a keyboard with a numeric keypad (as most people do), then you should move your chair slightly to the right when using the mouse intensively. The smaller the distance between the mouse and your stomach, the less strain is put on your right arm and shoulder.

Technique

Warming-up

Each day your arms/fingers perform an outstanding amount of work. Rub your hands together at least before starting to work in the morning and after returning from lunch. Shake out your arms vigorously and move your shoulders forward and backward in small circles. In the acute pain phase, I found long-sleeved shirts helpful. When I wore t-shirts, I put arm sleeves on to keep my underarms warm.

Finger movements while typing

Real 10-finger touch typing may be efficient, but it's not necessarily ergonomic! The faster you move your fingers, the more you strain your finger tendons and underarm muscles. In severe RSI cases it may be advisable to move the whole arm up and down while typing.

The advantage of 10-finger touch typing - an equal distribution of the load on all fingers - is often destroyed by a rigid arm position and far splayed out fingers. So if you use all 10 fingers, then please move the entire forearm while typing (less splaying out of fingers) and reduce your overall speed. Complicated keyboard shortcuts should be executed with two hands.

Regardless of how many fingers you use, always apply only the minimum pressure necessary.

Keyboard shortcuts

Various keyboard shortcuts can make your life easier by reducing the number of mouse clicks or keystrokes for certain actions. Most programs show those combinations in the menu bar next to the corresponding entry. Many programs use the same combinations, so you will have internalized the basics after a short period. If the two keys don't lie next to each other, please use both hands.

"Normal"	Shortcut	Description
Right-click > Cut	Ctrl + X	Cuts the selected text / object
Right-click > Copy	Ctrl + C	Copies the selected text / object
Right-click > Paste	Ctrl + V	Inserts the selected text / object
Edit > Undo	Ctrl + Z	Undo the last action
Edit > Redo	Ctrl + Y	Reverse an undo command
Multiple keystrokes (arrow keys)	Ctrl + Arrow key	Moves the cursor before / behind a word
Multiple keystrokes (delete / backspace)	Ctrl + Del / Backspace	Deletes a word (Del = behind the mouse cursor, Backspace = before)
Scrolling with the mouse	Page up	Scrolls up one page
Scrolling with the mouse	Page down	Scrolls down one page
Arrow keys or clicking with the mouse	Pos1	Document: Moves the cursor to the beginning of the current line; Website: Jumps to the top of the page
Arrow keys or clicking with the mouse	End	Document: Moves the cursor to the end of the current line; Website: Jumps to the bottom of the page
Drag the scrollbar with the mouse	Ctrl + Pos1	Moves the cursor to the beginning of a document
Drag the scrollbar with the mouse	Ctrl + End	Moves the cursor to the end of a document
Highlight with the mouse	Ctrl + Shift + Arrow	Highlights a word

"Normal"	Shortcut	Description
	key	
Highlight with the mouse	Shift + Pos1	Highlights everything from the cursor position to the beginning of the current line
Highlight with the mouse	Shift + End	Highlights everything from the cursor position to the end of the current line
Double-click on "My Computer" (this icon is usually only available on the desktop)	Win + E	Opens the Explorer
View > Refresh or - if available - by clicking on a special button in the menu bar	F5	Refreshes the current view (Explorer, Internet Explorer, Firefox etc.)
Left-click on a program in the taskbar	Alt + Tab	Switches between open windows (you can hold Alt and press the Tab key several times)

Move your arm instead of your wrist

If the pain primarily affects your wrist, use your entire arm to move the mouse. The same can be applied to the keyboard: don't spread your fingers unnaturally to reach keys lying further out, but simply move your arm.

Switch mouse arm

Spread the stress of the mouse on both hands. All recommended ergonomic mice (see Equipment, page 29) have a USB interface, so you can connect two mice simultaneously. As a right-hander I needed one week to be able to operate a mouse with my left hand.

Reduce double-click speed and/or single-click to open an item

Lower the strain of your index finger by reducing the double-click speed.

Windows: Start > Control Panel > Mouse > Double-click speed

For many actions you can also simply press the Enter key instead of one double-click (e.g. open a file).

Files in the Explorer and desktop shortcuts can be opened with a simple left-click instead of a double-click. To activate this option open the Explorer > Tools > Folder Options > General > Single-click to open an item (point to select).

Use auto click program

An auto click program enables clickless use of the computer. The software performs a mouse click after a certain time of inactivity (usually 0,5 - 1 second). It works with any other program.

- ... ЪI AutoClick (free)[1]
  ...лClick (paid)[2]
  ...NOME): Dwell Click Setting[3]

Regular breaks /alternation

To counteract monotonous office work, it is advised to take many micro-breaks instead of just one longer break. This means that when you work intensively, you should shake out your hands every 5 minutes and get up at least every half an hour (go to the copier, make coffee, make phone calls while standing, stretch your arms ...). Even if you are determined to obey these break schedules, you will probably miss a lot of the breaks. Software which reminds you to take regular breaks is of great help.

- Windows: Workrave (free)[4]
- Mac: AntiRSI (paid)[5] / Stretch (paid)[6]
- Linux: Break Timer (free)[7]

You should try to plan ahead your workday in a way that monotonous PC work is interrupted by other types of activities (e.g. client meetings, internal meetings, literature study).

A very common mistake is to rest the hand on the mouse, even when you actually don't use it. The same applies to the keyboard. As long as you don't use any of your input devices, place your hands comfortably in your lap. And avoid putting your bare forearms on cold surfaces.

Shake out your arms

Stand up, let your arms hang loosely beside your hips and shake them out.

Massage your arms

You can perform an arm massage on your own, which relaxes the muscles and helps prevent muscle stiffness.

---

1 http://artistdetective.com/rsiautoclick.htm
2 https://itunes.apple.com/de/app/dwellclick/id402414007
3 https://help.gnome.org/users/mousetweaks/stable/mouse-a11y-how-to-stop-features.html.en
4 http://www.workrave.org/
5 https://itunes.apple.com/de/app/antirsi/id442007571
6 https://itunes.apple.com/de/app/stretch/id658827081
7 https://launchpad.net/brainbreak

Hot / cold water (contrast baths)

Immerse your forearms 10-15 seconds in hot, and after that in cold water. That can be repeated multiple times to stimulate blood circulation.

Don't try out all of the tips at the same time. Start with one recommendation and implement another each day. Please don't give up too early. Give yourself at least two weeks to become accustomed.

If you don't have RSI symptoms, don't be concerned after reading this book. Always remember: millions of people work on the PC every day and in most cases won't develop pain. As long as you follow a few basic rules (regular breaks etc.), there is a high chances that you will be spared from RSI.

Stretching exercises

Due to our daily work our muscles shorten and become stiff. With stretching we can reduce muscle tension and maintain or restore the original range of motion. Although the stretching exercises for the forearms are most important, you should also perform all other exercises regularly, because the entire upper body is affected by non-ergonomic working positions.

Please don't overdo it in the first few days. No (additional) pain should appear. If you haven't used your hands for an extended period of time and have possibly even worn wrist splints, then it will take at least a week before any improvement might be felt. My wrist pain became significantly worse after the first two days, so I had to take a break again. From the second week onwards I felt a slight improvement almost after each stretch.

In acute RSI cases, you should perform all exercises 2-3 times a day for about 15-20 seconds each (unless indicated otherwise). Even if you only have problems with one hand, you should still perform all the exercises with both sides. Throughout the day you will need about 30-45 minutes in total. As prevention it is sufficient if you perform all exercises just once daily *(see treatment plans, page 20)*. It is better to hold a stretch longer and make fewer iterations, than to hold it shorter and do more iterations.

At first I did all stretching exercises sequentially (with the help of a list of all exercises), and then started to work. By the time I had internalized most stretches, I was able to flexibly integrate them into my workday. This also helps with the regular PC breaks. But don't pressure yourself with all those stretching exercises! If you forget some of them at times, that won't make a huge difference. Also there is no fixed order, rotate the sequence.

With sensory disturbances, numbness or tingling in the hands or arms, you should have a look at the chapter *Passive stretching exercises (page 48)* as well.

This book is designed to provide helpful information on the subjects discussed. It is not meant to be used, nor should it be used, to diagnose or treat any medical condition. For diagnosis or treatment of any medical problem consult your own physician and discuss the content of this book with him/her.

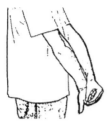 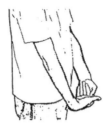 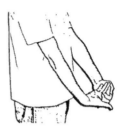

With straight arms, hold both hands in front of your hip area and bend the wrists to the right (palms facing up). Now you embrace the four fingers of your right hand with your left hand and pull it up (figure 1). After ten seconds, you rotate the right hand by almost 180° and stop again for ten seconds (figure 2). Finally, turn it forward as far as possible (figure 3). Repeat this exercise with the other hand. Make sure not to pull up your shoulders during the exercise

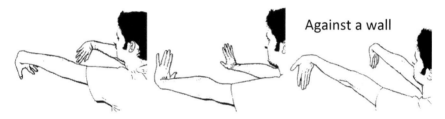

Against a wall

Lean against a wall with your arms straight. Rotate the hands inwards as far as possible, hold for ten seconds (figure 1). Then turn them upwards, without lifting them from the wall. Hold for another ten seconds (figure 2). Finally rotate your hands outwards as far as possible (figure 3).

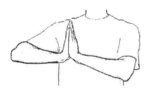

Press your palms against each other and slide both arms in one direction (right or left). Hold this position for at least 20 seconds and slide your arms in the other direction then.

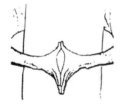

Splay out your fingers and press the fingertips of both hands against each other.

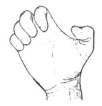

Make a fist and then open the hand very slowly (ten seconds) while trying to hold all fingers in a flexed position.

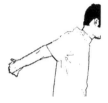

Interlace your hands behind your back and pull both arms upward.

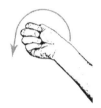

Hold your arm straight, make a fist with your thumb inside and tilt your hand slightly downward.

This exercise consists of eight different head positions. Each one should be performed for about ten seconds:

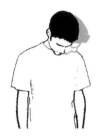

1. Forward
2. In the direction of the armpit
3. To the side (towards the shoulder)
4. Backward
5. Backward & to the side

Positions two, three and five each to the right and left.

To enhance the stretching effect, you can gently pull the opposite arm down.

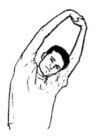

Hold your arms above your head and bend your upper body to one side.

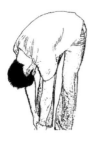

Bend your upper body forward and hold for about 10 seconds. Twist your upper body a little bit and hold again.

Against a wall

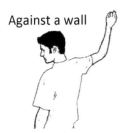

Standing sideways against a wall, lean against it with your forearm (elbow joint greater than 90°) and push your upper body slightly forward. The stretch should be felt in the chest/armpit area.

Against a wall

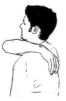

Place one arm on the opposite shoulder and lean against a wall, touching it just with your elbow.

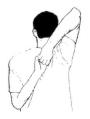

Try to hook your hands behind your back. If that doesn't work for you, you can also push down the upper elbow (right arm in the image) with the other arm.

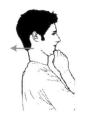

Pull the head back and hold for 10 seconds. Subsequently push the chin lightly back some more with your hand and hold again.

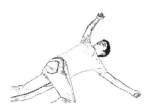

Lying on the floor

Lie on your back, slide one leg over the other, pull the elevated knee to a 90° angle and press it on the ground lightly. In extension of the straight leg, raise one arm and try to press it on the ground (in the most uncomfortable position). After a minute slowly unwind yourself and repeat the exercise with the other leg/arm.

Passive stretching exercises

Sensory disturbances, numbness or tingling in the arms or hands may indicate a nerve related problem. The nerves of the arm originate from the cervical vertebrae and run between collarbone and ribs into the arm (right picture). When using the computer, people often sit in a slightly forward-leaning posture. This reduces the free space below the collarbone and puts pressure on the nerves and blood vessels running between collarbone and ribs. This is the most common form of the so-called Thoracic Outlet Syndrome[1,2].

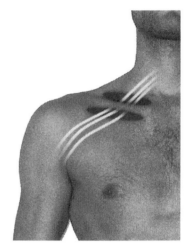

Often the *active stretching exercises (page 43)* are sufficient to eliminate minor complaints. The three most important exercises are shown in the image on the right (the third exercise with the head tilted back).

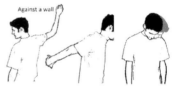

If there is no improvement, you can stretch the dark area above and below the collarbone with your fingers or a rounded, elongated object (e.g. a massage stick). Try to apply pressure to the area behind the collarbone for at least ten seconds. Slightly move the arm to find the most effective position. In the beginning, you should seek help from a physical therapist. This stretch for me was the only measure that resulted in an immediate and significant improvement. The uncomfortable feeling to "sense" my forearm all the time went away. Although this kind of numbness often came back after a few hours or days, the symptom-free periods between the stretches became longer and longer.

Surgery is possible in exceptional cases. Please consult a doctor.

---

1 http://en.wikipedia.org/wiki/Thoracic_outlet_syndrome
2 http://www.nismat.org/ptcor/thoracic_outlet

Trigger point massage

Definition

Trigger points are adhesions of muscle fibers with its surrounding connective tissue (called fascia). They can cause pain in other areas of the body (referred pain). They often dissolve after some time or they are too small to cause lasting discomfort. However, after working in a non-ergonomic posture for years, those trigger points can get very painful. Trigger points can occur in any muscle and cause pain in almost any area of the body. Head, neck and back pain is a common result.

Treatment

The actual muscle trigger points are not painful in a normal state. But they can be felt as a "knot" or stiff point by yourself or by a third party (e.g. physical therapist). Less pronounced trigger points cannot always be clearly identified.

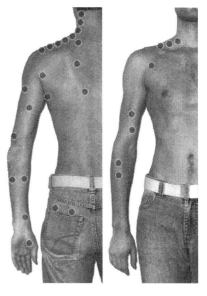

You can massage all trigger points shown on this page with your fingertips or palm of your hand in circular movements applying gentle pressure. You should feel an uncomfortable pressure pain. Since under pressure the knot often wobbles to one side, you have to constantly reposition your finger. To cope with trigger points on the back, you can lie down on a hard surface with your back on two tennis balls.

You might also have trigger points which are difficult to identify. I recommend professional help in the form of a physical therapist (especially at the start and if both your arms are affected).

You can massage the trigger points every two days and after that you should perform a round of *stretching exercises (page 43)*. After two to three weeks the referred pain should slowly subside.

Tools

Recent research findings state that elastic fascia is an extremely important part in the prevention of injuries. Even if you don't have any trigger points yet, you should train your fascia. For one thing this is done by regular stretching and for another thing by massages. Professional massages are most effective, but are also very expensive in the long term. I want to introduce you to two relatively cheap tools that I use regularly:

Tapping massager

Most office workers have painful spots on the upper back, so you should massage this area regularly, even if you can't identify trigger points. The best solution I found is a "tapping massager".[1] It sounds like a ridiculous product promoted by a home shopping channel, but it does work for me! I use it at least once a week and my neck and upper back pain is completely gone.

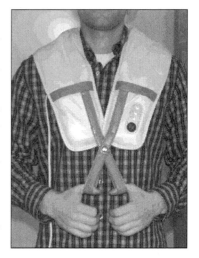

Some other reviewers criticize the following aspects, which I want to respond to:

- "It is too strong." - The massager has 10 different intensity levels. If level 1 is too strong for you, you should wear a sweater or put a towel between the device and your back. After a couple of uses, your muscles will become softer and level 1 won't feel too strong any more. I use it on level 10 and it just feels great!
- "After 15 minutes it switches itself off." - Yes it does, but 15 minutes should be long enough for one person. Another reason is, that it gets quite warm (which is very pleasant while using) and has to cool down a bit. Wait 5 minutes and it's good to go another round of 15 minutes.
- "The massage is only performed on two spots." - You can adjust the height of those spots by lowering the device. You can reach all muscles left and right of your spine from the neck down to your lower back.

---

1 http://www.amazon.com/gp/product/B0053UPAYS/

Foam roller

With a foam roller you can release adhesions and muscle stiffness. In contrast to the tapping massager, which you can use passively, the use of a foam roller is much more strenuous. I recommend it from *phase 3 (page 25)* in combination with the tapping massager. There are several brands available, I recommend *The Grid Foam Roller* or the *Blackroll*. They are of good quality and you receive a couple of exercises in the package. You should avoid those exercises which involve straining your hands (instead, support your body weight with your forearms). The exercises 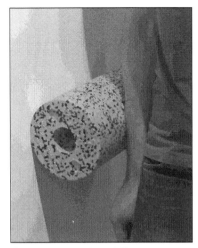 shown can be easily combined with my *strengthening program (page 54)*

The two most important exercises for your forearms can be seen in this video.[1] With the help of your body, you can apply exactly the amount of pressure which is pleasant for you.

1 https://www.youtube.com/watch?v=jSwC8Cby2zs

Nerve mobilization

Sensory disturbances, numbness and tingling in the arms are signs that the nerves are irritated somewhere on the way from the spine to the fingertips. One reason might be a spinal disc herniation, although that's not common for RSI sufferers. However if you have any of the symptoms mentioned, please have a neurologist or orthopedist look at your case. Only if other serious diseases have been ruled out, you can start with the exercises shown in this chapter.

With the exercises shown below, you can gently move the affected nerves in their sheaths back and forth. Light complaints can be resolved in a few days or weeks. If you have stronger nerve irritation, you might not notice any improvement, your pain might even get worse. In any case start very carefully and make only slight movements during the first few days. If you perform the exercises correctly, you will feel a slight pull in the entire arm to the fingertips. Nerves are very sensitive. If you overdo it, they can give you several days of pain.

Please have a look at the chapter *Treatment plans (page 25)* to find out if these nerve mobilization exercises suit your personal stage of the recovery.

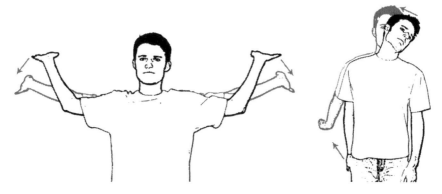

Form a "U" with your upper arms, palms facing upward. From this starting position stretch your arms slowly (image 1, arrows), hold a few seconds and go back to the starting position. Repeat this exercise five times. Return to the starting position, however this time with the tips of your fingers facing towards your head. Repeat five times.

The second exercise begins with your arms hanging down and your head tilted to the side. Tilt your opposite hand backward (palm facing up) and move that arm slightly to the back (image 2, bottom arrow). At the same time return your head back to the normal position (image 2, top arrow). Hold briefly and then move back to the starting position. Make sure you don't raise your shoulders. Repeat the exercise five times with each arm.

Strengthening

Strengthening exercises for chronic RSI

If you have/had a chronic form of RSI (six months or more) strengthening exercises are important for restoring the former muscle power. But if you start too early or too excessively, you could act counterproductively. **If you are still in constant pain, it's definitely too early!** After you have done the exercises shown in the other chapters for several weeks, your complaints should have at least temporarily improved. Now you can slowly begin to strengthen your upper body, because strong muscles can handle repetitive tasks better.

As a start, you should swim twice a week, so you build a solid foundation. You should avoid breaststroke because the hyperlordosis might amplify neck and back problems. Backstroke and crawl are preferred. Depending on your fitness level, you can add the exercises listed here 2-4 weeks later (every two to three days, see *Treatment plans, page 25*). The first two weeks you should start easily and see what your body tolerates. Over time, you might find some exercises are too easy. Then you can increase the repetitions, extend the holding time or do a second round.

Especially exercises in which some of the body weight lies on the hands were unimaginable for me in the first few months. Please only do the exercises that you can perform without pain. Even after more than six months with the basic exercises I could not hold my body weight for pull-ups. Begin carefully and gradually try more exercises. "The more the better" is NOT what you should strive for. Overstressing your body could set you back several weeks, do not take any risk!

Strengthening exercises for mild discomforts

Athletically trained people have a lower risk of developing RSI[1], they profit from the increased endurance of their muscles. If you only have mild pain and you want to enter directly into phase four, you should initially focus solely on stretching exercises and other measures. Only after seeing an improvement should you start with strengthening exercises.

Risks

Many people do not always use the appropriate muscles for certain motions, but (unconsciously) compensate with adjacent muscles. The stronger the

1 ef. Ratzlaff, Charles R. et al. (2007). Work-related repetitive strain injury and leisure-time physical activity. Arthritis Care & Research. Volume 57, Issue 3: 495 - 500

muscles are, the longer you won't feel any pain. But especially those adjacent muscles, which do most of the work, might fail at some point. In this case, you will not be able to restore the normal state with these strengthening exercises; you might even make the situation worse!

Hence I advise you to show this chapter to a good physical therapist. He/she will watch you closely doing all exercises and can correct the execution if necessary. Since no body and not every problem is the same, he/she might be able to show you additional exercises, specially tailored for you.

Execution

It is important that you perform the exercises correctly. It would be counterproductive to use too much additional weight. Stick to the comments and continue breathing. Always keep your body tension. Otherwise you would stress your ligaments and tendons, without having a training effect for your muscles.

Muscles do not grow while performing an exercise, but only some time later in the resting phase (supercompensation). Every muscle needs a different amount of time to fully regenerate. As a rule of thumb: rest for 48 hours after each round of strengthening exercises.

Unless otherwise indicated, static exercises should be held for about 15 seconds for each side. Dynamic exercises should be repeated at least 7 times. One round of exercises with short breaks will take you 20 to 30 minutes.

Some of the exercises can be conducted with a foam roller (see *Trigger point massage, page 49*). In addition to strengthening your body, you are then training your fascia at the same time.

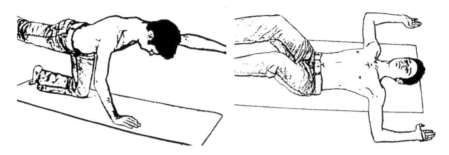

Core strengthening 1: In the neutral position you kneel on the floor and have both hands on the floor as well (arms straight). Knee, hip and shoulder joints are located at a 90° angle. Keep your head and neck in line with your spine and look down. Now lift one leg and the opposite arm, so that they form a horizontal line. Hold this position and then switch sides.

Core strengthening 2 (1-2 minutes): Lie on your back, legs still on the ground and keep your arms in a U-position (90°, see image). Press the entire body in line with your elbows down on the floor (at each point with the same force). Hold this position briefly. In addition try to press your entire spine evenly against the floor. Hold this position for 15-20 seconds. Now lift both legs and pull them up to a 90° angle. Push them slightly forward, with your spine still on the floor (see image).

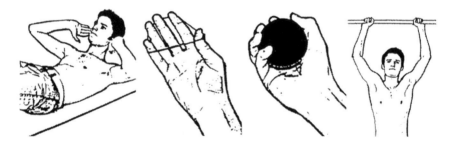

Crunches: Lie on your back with your knees bent. Lift your upper back slightly off the ground and stay in this position for a few seconds. Then lower your upper body slowly to the starting position. Repeat this exercise six times. The further you move your hands towards your head, the more difficult the exercise will become. Do not pull your head with your hands!

You should do another round for your oblique muscles: raise your upper body slightly to the right. Repeat right and left each six times.

Finger extensors: Spread your fingers against the resistance of a rubber band.

Forearm and hand strengthening: A gyroscopic exerciser is a tennis-ball sized gyroscope which is powered by circular wrist motions. Despite its low weight, it feels like lifting dumb bells. The faster you spin the mass inside the shell, the more difficult it becomes.

Pull-ups: Proper pull-ups can only be recommended as prevention *(phase 5, page 28)*. You can individually reduce the strain by supporting your body weight with your feet.

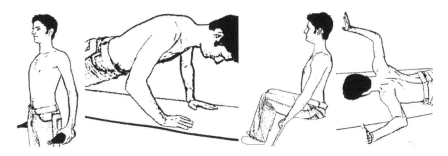

Shoulder strengthening 1: Take a bottle of water in each hand and circle your shoulders slowly backwards.

Pushups: Like pull-ups, pushups are only for prevention. To reduce the load, you can put your knees on the ground instead of your feet.

Core strengthening 3: Sit on the edge of a bed and lift your feet a few centimeters off the ground. Keep your back straight.

Shoulder strengthening 2: Lie on your stomach and lift your head slightly, without kinking the neck. Move your arms slowly up and down in each of the following positions:

a) Arms lying alongside your body (back of the hands facing up)

b) Arms to the side (thumbs up). Maximize the distance between both hands so that your shoulder blades stay apart.

c) Arms in U-position (hands upwards, see image).

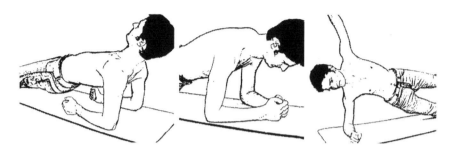

Back plank: Legs and torso form a straight line.

Front plank: The front plank is the wrist-friendly alternative to pushups. Legs and torso form a straight line.

Side plank: Legs and torso form a straight line. You can also put the upper arm alongside your body.

Psyche

As described in the chapter *Causes (page 6)*, the psyche may play a role in RSI in three different ways:

1. As a "concomitant": When you are in constant pain you might become afraid of your future and a pain memory develops. Please read the general section of this chapter from *work attitude* onwards.

2. As a trigger: Subliminal, severe stress (Tension Myositis Syndrome)

3. As a trigger: Fear of RSI

TMS (Tension Myositis Syndrome)

As an introduction to this issue please read the TMS-section in the chapter *Causes (page 8)*. The treatment strategy has similarities to erasing the pain memory, so that the following section should be of interest to all people who are in persistent pain. In return, all TMS sufferers should also look at the information about the *pain memory (page 66)*.

Inner tension, repressed problems or life changes can be the cause of your pain. TMS is not always the sole cause, it can also occur in addition to a physical overload. Pain can occur in any body part, but it often does where you expect pain. With the pain your brain tries to distract you from dealing with a (sometimes positive) life change. Due to the pain you might develop fear of using the affected body part because you don't want to aggravate the pain. You are caught in a vicious circle between a relieving posture and brain induced further pain.

To escape this vicious circle, have a look at the following strategy:

1. For one day engage yourself in the topic of TMS and read the respective success stories.[1] You will automatically gain euphoria that will help you in the early days. A pain-free life is possible!

2. Accept Dr. Sarno's theory. Yes, initially it is very difficult to believe that a real pain can be controlled by the brain alone and that there must not be any physical injury present. However, you have to really believe in it - be a 100% convinced. Give this theory a chance and try it out for a week, you have nothing to lose! Only if you then feel no improvement at all, your RSI is probably caused by a physical strain.

---

1 http://www.rsipain.com/other-personal-stories.php

3. Dr. Sarno recommends patients with a clear TMS diagnosis to stop all stretching exercises etc., because the pain is not caused by a physical overload which can be counteracted with appropriate exercises. All exercises would only draw unnecessary attention to the existing pain and would be counterproductive. If your diagnosis is very clear (you were not exposed to repeated stress over a longer period of time), then you should stop other exercises in this phase. If you're not sure if the Tension Myositis Syndrome is the sole cause, then I recommend you perform at least a few stretching exercises. With those few stretches you will counteract the following thought you will inevitably develop during the week: "Am I not just wasting my time? Shouldn't I perform conventional exercises instead?" If you do both, you create a win-win situation. If the pain is (at least partly) caused psychologically, then you are on track of becoming pain free after this week (the first step is the most difficult). If you don't feel any improvement, then at least you haven't lost any time.

4. Create a list of things that affect your feelings (even supposedly positive ones). Possible areas are:

    a. Adverse childhood experiences (very strict rules, abuse, problems of your parents [alcohol, drugs, depression], separation of parents ...)

    b. Personality traits (you want to make it right for everyone, perfectionism, low self-esteem ...)

    c. Current personal challenges/problems (serious illness or death of a family member or friend, divorce, debt, problems with work colleagues or friends, new boss, new job, partner starts/quits an employment, legal dispute, feelings of shame, feelings of guilt, vacation, relocation, marriage, pregnancy, birth of a child ...)

    d. Trivial matters that always bothered you, but you have never addressed (attitude towards certain topics or behavior in certain situations from your partner or from friends)

    e. Your own age and thoughts about the inevitable death

5. Each day choose a different theme and write down everything you can think of. Write about your feelings and consider various strategies to address the problems. This regular work requires some time and effort, but it is currently the most effective method of treating TMS. According to Dr.

Sarno about 20% of his patients need psychotherapeutic help to overcome their traumatic events. When in doubt, take up professional help.

6. Read your records regularly and work constantly to implement your strategies. Work on yourself and discuss unpleasant topics with your family and friends. Something that you or others cannot change, you must try to accept. You will not be able to clear up every little annoyance. It is enough to identify it clearly and to accept your feelings. For example: you think that a family member acts embarrassingly in public. Previous talks couldn't bring any improvement. That you are ashamed of another person is not a bad thing. However it becomes stressful for you if you feel uncomfortable and embarrassed to be ashamed. This is perfectly natural, stand by your feelings and do not try to suppress them.

7. Your muscles aren't overloaded and the tissue isn't damaged! Start slowly with everyday activities and try to use your hands normally. Also apply the tactics for erasing the *pain memory (page 66)*. When you see an initial success, restart light computing tasks and increase the time continuously.

Additional information can be found in the book *The Mind Body Prescription*[1] by Dr. Sarno (who has come up with the term Tension Myositis Syndrome) as well as on numerous websites[2].

Fear of RSI

1. If you work **less than 2 hours a day** on a PC (and are not exposed to comparable repetitive motions): your risk is very limited. Follow the instructions in the *Summary (page 23)*, but continue to work as usual. You can also have a look at the *Treatment plans (section "prevention", page 28)*.

2. If you work **more than 2 hours a day** on a PC (or are exposed to comparable repetitive motions): even if you are at risk, you really don't need to be afraid! As long as you follow the tips of this book (equipment, breaks, stretching ...) your risk of developing RSI is reduced dramatically. You can find an overview with all tips in the chapter *Treatment plans (page 25)*. Particularly in stressful work phases you should take regular, short breaks and shake out your arms. Whenever you think that you just don't have the time to pause for a few seconds and only want to quickly complete a task, it is time for a short break! There is software available you can install on your computer which reminds you to take regular breaks *(page 41)*. Millions of

1 Sarno, John E. (1999). The Mindbody Prescription: Healing the Body, Healing the Pain. New York: Warner Books
2 http://www.rsipain.com/links.php

people work in extremely non-ergonomic positions and don't develop any pain. If you follow the basic advice you are quite save.

Work attitude

Very diligent people who take on voluntary extra work and skip breaks are especially prone to Repetitive Strain Injuries. If you belong to this group and develop pain, you will probably want to continue to work as usual.

Right here you have to step in, because the sooner you address the pain, the faster you will be able to work normally again. Discuss the problem with your partner, your boss and your colleagues. They all need to know that you need to take your time temporarily and must adhere to regular short breaks. You should be as transparent as possible in order to counteract any additional outside pressure ("What funny exercises is he/she doing?" "Is that a mouse for disabled people?" "Sick of PC work? You only want to work less!").

You also have to work on your work attitude:

1. Accept your disease! You don't benefit from continuing to work for another two months in pain, if that results in being unable to work properly for the rest of your life.

2. Draw the right conclusions and change your behavior. This is also in the interest of your employer. He will not want to trade a single completed project with the subsequent loss of your work force.

3. You cannot please everyone 100% of the time; this is a fact and cannot be changed! Don't be frustrated, you have done your best.

Work organization

With sophisticated self-organization you can work more efficiently. A reduced workload does not necessarily mean that you also achieve significantly less. The first pain often occurs in a very stressful situation. For example when a project must be completed by the end of the month and you have to do a lot of overtime in the last week. A realistic time schedule and a list of priorities would have made more sense.

The Pareto principle states that 80% of the result is achieved in only 20% of the time. The remaining 80% of the time is consumed for only 20% of the result. For perfectionists (a 100% result) it does not matter if they start with the unimportant tasks and then finally work on the most important parts.

However, this approach is very inefficient. A good result (95%) could be achieved in significantly less time. In practice this means that at the beginning of each project you should create a sort list of all sub-goals in order of importance. After about 20% of the estimated time all indispensable tasks will already be done and now you can devote the rest of your available time on the less important tasks. If the original schedule turns out to be too tight, you have two options:

1. Nocturnal overtime for a 100% result (if you are a perfectionist you want it that way - people without a priority list have to work overtime, as they have not even started an important sub-task)

2. Achieve a 95% result within normal working hours and without stress due to your priority list.

Here is an example of a small task (creating a presentation):

Priority	Description	Scheduled time	Time in %
Elementary	Work out the content of the presentation	2,0	
Elementary	Create slides	0,5	22
Very important	Define slide transitions	0,5	
Very important	Create charts	1,0	
Very important	Practice lecture	2,0	30
Important	Revise texts	1,0	
Important	Check spelling	0,5	
Important	Refine layout	1,0	22
Optional	Create animations	1,0	
Optional	Create handout	1,0	
Optional	Create opening and closing slides	0,5	
Optional	Print out slides, in case the projector is defective	0,5	26
		11,5	100

With this example you can see that you have already achieved a good result in half the scheduled time (priority elementary and very important). A presentation would be possible now. The rest of the time you can spend on improvements that are desirable, but which could also be omitted if time is tight.

If you hadn't worked according to a priority list (and started with the layout, animations, opening and closing slides etc.), you would probably be stressed towards the end. Any unforeseen "emergency" would have also jeopardized the timely finishing.

The following additional points can also result in a significant workload reduction:

1. Delegate tasks

2. Practice saying "No!" (don't undertake all tasks which could also be done by someone else)

3. Don't postpone unpleasant tasks

4. Perform routine tasks such as responding to e-mails during mid-afternoon energy slumps

5. Only budget 60% of your working time for fixed tasks

6. Set concrete and realistic goals:
   An example:
   What: Reduce strains in the workplace
   How: Take 10-seconds short breaks
   Extend: Every 10 minutes
   Period: 4 weeks
   "To reduce strains in the workplace, I'll take short 10-second breaks every 10 minutes. After four weeks, I will check if I have achieved my goal with this measure."

Will I recover?

RSI is a vicious circle: the greater the pain, the less you want to use your hands. In extreme cases, they are put in casts. When the complaints are finally gone after weeks, months or even years, the muscles have degenerated to the extent that you can't properly perform even the simplest activities. Even everyday work on the computer is no longer possible. The person affected will probably question the ability to be able to ever use their hands again (at least I thought that way). Although apparently one has done everything possible, even light work will be painful. At this point, it is very important not to give up. You can be healthy again! Of course, in the early days your arms are not nearly as strong as they used to be, but the muscles can be rebuilt with light *strengthening exercises (page 54)*.

The road to recovery is like a roller coaster ride. There will be days with no pain and others where your hands will feel as bad as in the beginning. At first you will only have a few painless hours a week, but over time those painless hours will return on a daily basis. After a few weeks you will have more good than bad phases and you will be symptom-free in the end.

In addition to this development, the intensity of my pain remained the same at first, which was very frustrating. Only over time, as the good phases outweighed the bad, the pain intensity slowly decreased.

Psychological consequences of long-term RSI

The longer you have problems with a repetitive strain injury, inevitably the more your mind plays a role. You probably will not be able to pursue your recreational activities (volleyball, tennis, hockey, windsurfing, violin, piano ...) and therefore you will also meet less with friends. If you stay home alone, then you will probably often think of all the negative consequences of RSI. "How nice it would be if I could do ... now." From my own experience I know that over time one loses the desire to do anything at all. "Maybe it will hurt my arms. I'd rather do nothing, than do something wrong ..."

Especially in temporary bad phases, please consider the following:

1. Accept your illness. Do not take it as an "excuse" that you have to sit at home and cannot do what you enjoy. Continue doing your usual activities that you can perform without putting excessive strain on your hands (cinema, theater, swim, jog ...).

2. See your situation as an opportunity for something new. You've probably wanted to start something but then discarded it due to time constraints. Or you cultivate an existing talent. Now is the time! (jog, swim, sing, read books, magazines and specialist journals, learn a foreign language ...).

3. You will be healthy again! Read other personal stories of former RSI sufferers.[1] Particularly in the very bad phases it will help you overcome bad moods.

4. If you, your family or friends think that you cannot cope alone with your negative thoughts, then do not be afraid to get professional help. A visit to a psychologist is absolutely no shame! Many people do not dare to seek professional help because they are afraid of being considered insane or mentally confused. That's absolutely not true, most patients are ordinary people like you and me. Almost every one of us will go through a very

1 http://www.rsipain.com/other-personal-stories.php

difficult period at least once in his/her life and many will also consult a psychologist (it is usually just not talked about). You can only benefit!

Pain memory

When your muscles and tendons have completely regenerated and you can already do all normal household activities without problems, it might happen that the pain reoccurs immediately when doing computer work. This phenomenon is called pain memory. After a long time in pain (approx. 3 months) your brain automatically connects the computer work with pain, even if physical injuries are all healed. In order to "reprogram" your brain as quickly as possible, here are a few tips:

- Work for a few minutes on the computer every day, just quit shortly before the point at which the pain or discomfort usually occurs. It is very important that the pain threshold is **not** exceeded and you stop consequently. Every day you extend the time by a few minutes. After two weeks you will notice that you will be able to work longer without pain compared to the first day. On days you have permanent pain even without working, don't switch on the PC that day. You can extend the pain-free phase by increasing blood flow to your arms *(page 68)*.

- Combine the computer activity with something pleasant, for example listening to your favorite CD.

- Give your hands a comprehensive sensory input, i.e. you regularly palpate small objects with your fingers (without looking at the object).

- Regularly work at the computer wearing thin gloves. The feeling when typing on the keyboard is a completely different one and helps the brain to erase the pain memory.

- From time to time type on various surfaces, e.g. on a wooden or glass table, on your lap, on a piece of paper. It is important that you move your fingers as if you were writing a correct sentence on your "virtual keyboard".

- Think of friends/colleagues who have never had RSI pain. Or think of LAN party attendees, who play PC games three days in a row. Without breaks. Without stretching exercises. In a non-ergonomic posture. The human body is capable of compensating extreme strain, you will be able to use the PC again without pain.

- Consider your pain as an object, with which you can talk. If pain shows up, talk to it (inside or out loud). Say that you understand that your brain tricks you. You know that the pain has no reason to exist and should therefore disappear. What might sound ridiculous really works in many cases! Try it out. You have to believe in it a 100%. You have nothing to lose! I promise you an incredible feeling when you experience it for the first time.

Additional treatment

Please have a look at the *Treatment plans (page 25)*, so you know when and what action is appropriate.

> This book is designed to provide helpful information on the subjects discussed. It is not meant to be used, nor should it be used, to diagnose or treat any medical condition. For diagnosis or treatment of any medical problem consult your own physician and discuss the content of this book with him/her.

Improve blood circulation

Since RSI is mainly due to a lack of blood flow, all circulation-promoting measures are positive. The following points will give you specific suggestions.

Jogging

Jogging regularly not only improves blood circulation, but also improves your fitness and general physical condition (which in turn is positive for the recovery of RSI). If your pain is still very strong, you can let your arms hang alongside the body while running.

Contrast baths

Fill two adjacent plastic tubs with hot and very cold water (if possible with ice cubes). Immerse both forearms in the hot tub for at least 3 minutes and then immediately put them into the cold water. After 15-20 seconds you start again with the hot water and then finish in the cold tub.

Simpler (but less effective) are contrast baths in the shower or in the sink. There is a recommended order: hot (right arm, from the hand to the shoulder, first the outside, then the inside), cold, hot, cold. Then the left arm.

After the last cold bath you should wear something with long sleeves and shake out the arms gently.

Sauna/steam bath

Sauna sessions stimulate blood circulation and in combination with a subsequent cold bath form a good vascular training.

Keep your forearms and hands warm

Wearing long sleeved clothing helps to keep your forearms and wrists warm. Alternatively you can wear thin gloves or arm warmers during the day and at night.

Rub your hands together

Rub your hands together quickly. The friction will warm your fingers and improve blood circulation.

Pump with your hands

Hold your arms up straight over your head and open and close your hands very quickly - for half a minute. Bend your upper body forward and then shake out your arms until all the blood is flowed back again.

Massage ball

At my workplace there is always a massage ball within reach. Firstly you can warm your hands with rotating movements, secondly it supresses the burning sensation in the forearms which sometimes occurs after prolonged keyboard work.

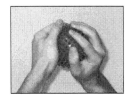

Swelling

In the early days of severe RSI cases forearms or wrists are prone to swelling. In this case, you should definitely go to the doctor to rule out other diseases or injuries. The only sensible time to fight RSI with immobilization (wrist brace) and anti-inflammatory tablets or creams is now - at the very beginning. If you wear wrist braces, you should not continue to wear them after the swelling has subsided, in order not to harm the mobility of the joints and your muscle strength. In exceptional cases, you can temporarily wear wrist braces in stressful situations (if they bring a significant reduction in pain).

In my experience most sufferers prefer cooling their swollen arms. After the swelling has subsided, heat is usually more pleasant (stimulate blood circulation, see above).

Relaxation techniques

A regular change between tension and relaxation is common and very useful. However, when longer periods of tension are not followed with sufficient times of relaxation, unhealthy stress develops. This can manifest itself in many ways, including headaches, impaired concentration, increased blood pressure, fatigue, aggression, insecurity and anxiety. Stressed people usually have an increased muscle tension, even if that is often not perceived by themselves. The heavily strained upper body muscles are unable to regenerate sufficiently in phases without workload.

The goal should be to not let stress determine your life. The basis for this is a good work organization. You can support reducing muscle tension by using relaxation techniques. Basically it is not so important which method you use (e.g. autogenic training, progressive muscle relaxation, qigong, yoga, biofeedback, meditation or hypnosis). You should use the technique which suits you best (or even a combination of several techniques). The more often a method is applied, the faster a relaxation can ensue. Even a break of a few minutes can then be used effectively.

A good introduction into the different techniques can be found at helpguide.org.[1]

Deep friction massage

With RSI the tendons in the elbow area may just be as sensitive to pressure as with tennis elbow. The special treatment (deep friction massage) which takes about two to four weeks is explained in the Chapter *Tennis elbow (page 72)* in detail.

Pain diary

Each RSI sufferer should continuously record important key data to fall back on when visiting a doctor so that you can reconstruct the development over a longer period. But you should not write a conventional pain diary and make an entry every day. The constant dealing with your own pain would be counterproductive for the healing process. Limit your entries in the acute pain phase to about one per week (later even rarer). Any significant change in pain intensity, duration of pain or location of pain should be noted down. You should also write down new treatments, medications or doctor's visits. In addition, you should note the maximum time that you can perform repetitive motions (e.g. PC work) without major pain.

The longer the pain persists, the more you start to question whether your body has started to heal at all. Often the intensity of the pain has only slightly decreased, but the pain occurs much less frequently and the time you spend on

---

1 http://www.helpguide.org/articles/stress/relaxation-techniques-for-stress-relief.htm

the computer each day has increased steadily. Without a pain diary, it is very difficult to understand how you felt several months ago.

The following table can be found as a document on my website[1].

Date	xx/xx/xx
Location and intensity of the pain	Severe pain on the inside of the left wrist Right forearm slightly numb
Duration of pain	Several hours a day, numbness mostly in the mornings
Treatment / medication	Started with stretching exercises (after consultation with orthopedist XY)
PC work with no major pain	30 minutes
Special activities / strains / miscellaneous	Driven for two hours today, no additional complaints

---

1 http://www.rsipain.com/pain-diary.docx

Tennis elbow

Definition

As written in the chapter *What is RSI? (page 3)*, "tennis elbow" is often used as a synonym for repetitive strain injury, mouse arm or for general pain in the forearm. In contrast to these diffuse diseases, tennis elbow is a diagnosis for a clearer pattern of pain. Tennis elbow refers to local irritation or inflammation of the outer elbow area (where the forearm tendons connect to the bone).

Synonyms

The corresponding technical term is called epicondylitis. It exists in the following two forms:

1. Lateral epicondylitis (tennis elbow): pain in the outer elbow area
2. Medial epicondylitis (golfer's elbow): pain in the inner elbow area

Tennis elbow is more widespread.

Symptoms / pain

Pain in the elbow area (outside or inside) initially only occurs while playing tennis or golf or while working by hand. After a few hours or by the next day, the pain is usually gone. If the workload is not temporarily scaled back or if you don't perform stretching exercises, the pain may becomes persistent. In some cases people can't even clench

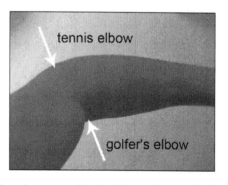

into a fist without severe pain and they have trouble holding objects of all kinds. The usually local pain in the elbow might radiate to the hand.

Causes

The cause is an overload of the affected tissue. However, many sufferers do not play too often but "only" have a poor technique. They grab the racket too forcefully, cramp in the game or play without warming up before.

A repetitive strain injury is not a classic tennis elbow! A tennis elbow usually arises from activities in which you hold something with a closed fist and you yourself are in motion. Repetitive strain injuries are caused by thousands of small finger/hand movements in a mostly non-ergonomic working posture. Although computer work can also cause tennis elbow, the tendinosis of the lateral epicondyle of the elbow then is usually just only one of several pain triggers. If you work at the computer several hours a day, the measures discussed in this chapter are very useful, but you can do much more! Please have a look at the chapter *Treatment plans (page 25)*.

Am I affected?

All those affected complain of a very painful spot at the elbow (tennis elbow: outside area, golfer's elbow: inside area, see pictures). The easiest way you can provoke the pain is by pulling your clenched hand in the direction of the arrow. The circle depicts the area where you should feel pain now. You can amplify the pain by either putting pressure on the circled area with your other hand or by pushing the other hand against the arrow.

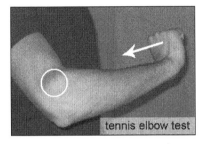

tennis elbow test

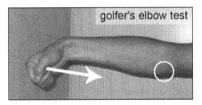

golfer's elbow test

This kind of pain mostly affects people over the age of 40, but as always, there are exceptions to that rule.

If you can see a (strong) swelling in the circled area, you might have bursitis. It might be the consequence of a hard impact or of reading with both elbows lying on a hard surface for several hours a day (and is then called "student's elbow"). In this case, the exercises in this chapter are not useful!

This book is designed to provide helpful information on the subjects discussed. It is not meant to be used, nor should it be used, to diagnose or treat any medical condition. For diagnosis or treatment of any medical problem consult your own physician and discuss the content of this book with him/her.

Therapy

Before you start with any exercise, you should wait until any existing swelling has subsided. You can support this process by cooling and with anti-inflammatory drugs (tablets and/or gels). Initially minimize the workload. Cortisone injections are not recommended because the risk of long term damage is high (especially when applied repeatedly) and an effect is often only short-lived. If your arms are swollen, you have to visit a doctor in any case!

Phase Treatment	1	2	3	4	5 Prevention
Treat swelling	X				
Minimize workload	X	X			
Stretching		X	X	X	X
Deep friction massage		X			
Myofascial release		X	X	X	X
Reduce workload		X	X		
Epicondylitis brace		X	X		
Work on sports technique		X	X		X
Warm up before exercise		X	X		X
Hanging				X	X

Stretching exercises

Stretching exercises are among the most effective treatments for tennis and golfer's elbow. The first exercise is primarily against a tennis elbow, the second and third are against a golfer's elbow. I recommend that you perform all three exercises no matter where your pain is located, because those three are the most important exercises against the repetitive strain injury. And with today's widespread use of computers, more and more people are diagnosed with this disease. In acute cases, you should perform all exercises 2-3 times a day. As prevention it is sufficient when you perform all exercises before and after stressful activities or at least once a day.

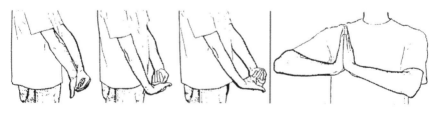

Left image: With straight arms, hold both hands in front of your hip area and bend the wrists to the right (palms facing up). Now you embrace the four fingers of your right hand with your left hand and pull it up (figure 1). After ten seconds, you rotate the right hand by almost 180° and stop again for ten seconds (figure 2). Finally, turn it forward as far as possible (figure 3). Repeat this exercise with the other hand. Make sure not to pull up your shoulders during the exercise.

Right image: Press your palms against each other and slide both arms in one direction (right or left). Hold this position for at least 20 seconds and slide your arms in the other direction then.

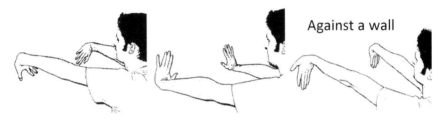

Against a wall

Lean against a wall with your arms straight. Rotate the hands inwards as far as possible, hold for ten seconds (figure 1). Then turn them upwards, without lifting them from the wall. Hold for another ten seconds (figure 2). Finally rotate your hands outwards as far as possible (figure 3).

Deep friction massage

Deep friction massage is a technique that forcefully massages the area where the forearm muscles are connected with tendons to the bone in the elbow area (humerus). The pressure causes additional micro injuries, which forces the body to immediately begin with repairing the tissue. Once the initial swelling has subsided, you can start with the deep friction massage. You can perform this massage yourself, but I recommend that you visit a physical therapist at least once so that he/she can show you how to do it correctly.

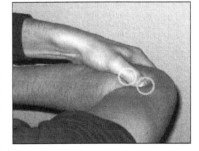

After a maximum of six massages you should feel an improvement, otherwise the treatment should be discontinued. A total of twelve treatments should not be exceeded. The deep friction massage can be applied two to three times a week for five minutes each. Rub your thumb back and forth over the painful tendon (in all directions). You have to find out the exact spot yourself, but it is usually near the areas of the circles on the photos. Although it is called a "massage", it doesn't feel like one. If you have a tennis or golfer's elbow, the deep friction massage will hurt! If it doesn't, you don't have tennis/golfer's elbow or you haven't found the correct spot yet.

In the subsequent repair phase, it is extremely important that you don't put your arm in plaster or permanently wear a wrist brace. The tissue has to be used lightly, in order to be able to regenerate properly. Light stretches are useful as well.

Myofascial release

The forearm muscles and their surrounding fascia (connective tissue) tend to stick together over time. Unlike the deep friction massage this myofascial release doesn't cause micro injuries. Thus it is much more pleasant to perform and should also be continued as means of prevention. Using a foam roller you can comfortably massage your forearms yourself *(see Trigger point massage, page 50)*.

Epicondylitis brace

When the deep friction massage and myofascial release bring about an effect, you can slowly resume your activity (usually a sport). An epicondylitis brace helps to reduce the stress on the tendon while playing. Do not forget to warm up before playing. Ideally you also work on your playing technique with a sports coach.

Hanging

When the pain has already subsided a bit, you can start hanging several times a day. Hanging means that you rest in a pull-up position for at least 30 seconds. If you don't have a stair for your hanging, you can use a doorway pull-up bar. You can start by hanging with your feet still on the ground to support your body weight. You don't have to do any pull-up, just hang with straight arms. With this exercise you also prevent back pain.

Healing period

Most sufferers will feel a significant improvement after four weeks of stretching exercises. However, mild pain can still occur several months later. A complete recovery usually occurs within six months.

Other treatment options

As prevention, you can strengthen your forearms with light strengthening exercises. This can be helped by a gyroscopic exerciser, a tennis-ball sized gyroscope which is powered by circular wrist motions. More exercises can be found in the chapter *Strengthening (page 54)*.

If all conventional treatments fail to improve your condition after several months, then there is the possibility of surgery (with all its risks).[1]

---

1 http://www.webmd.com/arthritis/surgery-for-tennis-elbow

Further information

Other personal stories

Unfortunately pain which accumulated over years cannot heal overnight; sufferers often fight for several weeks, months or even years. When setbacks occur during this time, one begins to doubt the ability of one's body to heal. Especially in these difficult times it is important not to lose a positive attitude. It helps immensely to read personal stories of former sufferers. I have therefore published other personal stories on my website.[1]

If you had problems with repetitive strain injury and you could significantly reduce the pain or are even symptom-free and want your healing strategies shared with other sufferers? Just write me an email (contact info is on my website) with your story, if you want it to be published there. Please write whether you want it to be published under your (fore)name or anonymously. If you have a website, feel free to insert a link into your story.

Your story could include:

- Type and location of the pain
- Time frame of the strain and (main) cause, e.g. Software developer for 15 years
- Treatment / medication
- Experiences with doctors
- Time frame of the pain
- Suggestions for activities with no or little hand use

---

1 http://www.rsipain.com/other-personal-stories.php

Health professionals

By popular demand, I created an online map[1] with health professionals (physicians/physical therapists/other RSI specialists) who know the condition RSI and should be able to treat it. I appreciate all your recommendations (contact info is on my website)!

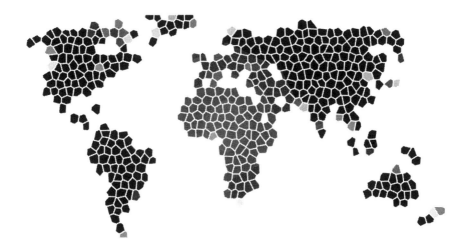

---

1 http://www.rsipain.com/health-professionals.php

Removable pages

On the following pages you will find the most important exercises, treatment plans and shortcuts in a compact overview. You can rip them out, so you do not always have to look into the book. The last page is a notice, which you are welcome to hang on the bulletin board of your school, university, company etc.

Everything is also available as PDF files on my website.[1]

Each of these little notes can be cut and stuck on your monitor as a reminder.

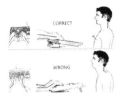

• Sit actively
• Take regular breaks
• Keep your elbows close to your waist

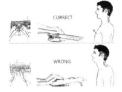

• Sit actively
• Take regular breaks
• Keep your elbows close to your waist

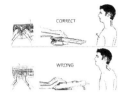

• Sit actively
• Take regular breaks
• Keep your elbows close to your waist

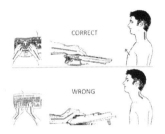

• Sit actively
• Take regular breaks
• Keep your elbows close to your waist

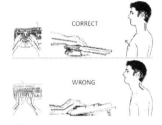

• Sit actively
• Take regular breaks
• Keep your elbows close to your waist

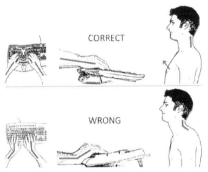

• Sit actively
• Take regular breaks
• Keep your elbows close to your waist

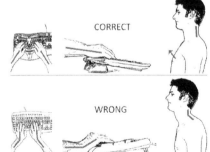

• Sit actively
• Take regular breaks
• Keep your elbows close to your waist

81

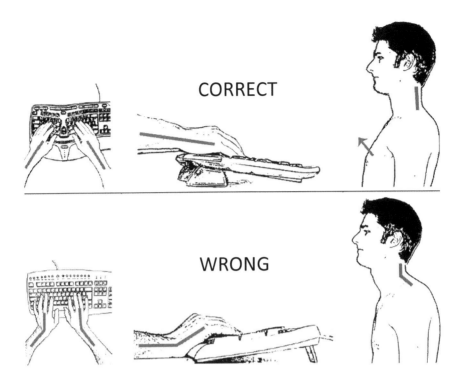

Sit actively

Do not remain in the same position for several hours, keep your body moving. If you are not currently using the keyboard or mouse, rest your hands in your lap.

Take regular breaks

Instead of having a few long breaks, take shorter breaks more often (shake out your hands and arms at least every five minutes, stand up every half an hour). Look out of the window at a distant object regularly to relax your eyes.

Keep your elbows close to your waist

The distance between your body and the keyboard should be minimal so that you do not have to reach out with your hands while typing. Keep your elbows close to your waist and the mouse next to the keyboard.

Use ergonomic equipment

Select from the wide range of ergonomic mice and keyboards. If possible, work on a height-adjustable desk and regularly use speech recognition software.

Phase / Treatment	1	2	3	4	5 Prevention
Ergonomic workplace (p. 29)	X	X	X	X	X
Work habits (p. 37) + Work attitude (p. 62)	X	X	X	X	X
Read other personal stories[1]	X	X	X	X	
Pain diary (p. 70)	X	X	X	X	
Treat swelling (p. 69)	X				
Minimize workload	X	X			
Reduce workload			X	X	
Erase pain memory (p. 66)			X	X	
Stimulate blood flow (p. 68)		X	X	X	X
Relaxation techniques (p. 69)		X	X	X	X
Deep friction massage (p. 75)			X		
Stretching (active p. 43 + passive p. 48)		X	X	X	X
Trigger point massage (p. 49)		X	X	X	X
Nerve mobilization (p. 52)			X	X	X
Strengthening (p. 54)				X	X

1 http://www.rsipain.com/other-personal-stories.php

Second phase

Monday	Tuesday	Wednesday	Thursday	Friday	Saturday	Sunday
	Running (at least 30 minutes)			Running (at least 30 minutes)		Running (at least 30 minutes)
Stretching	Stretching	Stretching	Stretching	Stretching	Stretching	Stretching
Trigger point massage		Trigger point massage			Trigger point massage	
Stretching	Stretching	Stretching	Stretching	Stretching	Stretching	Stretching
Relaxation techniques	Relaxation techniques	Relaxation techniques	Relaxation techniques	Relaxation techniques	Relaxation techniques	Relaxation techniques

Third phase

Monday	Tuesday	Wednesday	Thursday	Friday	Saturday	Sunday
	Running (at least 30 minutes)			Running (at least 30 minutes)		Swimming
Stretching	Stretching	Stretching	Stretching	Stretching	Stretching	Stretching
Trigger point massage	Nerve mobilization	Trigger point massage	Nerve mobilization		Trigger point massage	Nerve mobilization
	Deep friction massage			Deep friction massage		
Stretching	Stretching	Stretching	Stretching	Stretching	Stretching	Stretching
Erase pain memory	Erase pain memory	Erase pain memory	Erase pain memory	Erase pain memory	Erase pain memory	Erase pain memory
Relaxation techniques	Relaxation techniques	Relaxation techniques	Relaxation techniques	Relaxation techniques	Relaxation techniques	Relaxation techniques

Fourth phase

Monday	Tuesday	Wednesday	Thursday	Friday	Saturday	Sunday
	Running (at least 30 minutes)			Running (at least 30 minutes)		Swimming
Stretching	Stretching	Stretching	Stretching	Stretching	Stretching	Stretching
Trigger point massage	Nerve mobilization	Trigger point massage	Nerve mobilization		Trigger point massage	Nerve mobilization
	Strengthening			Strengthening		
Stretching	Stretching	Stretching	Stretching	Stretching	Stretching	Stretching
Erase pain memory	Erase pain memory	Erase pain memory	Erase pain memory	Erase pain memory	Erase pain memory	Erase pain memory
Relaxation techniques	Relaxation techniques	Relaxation techniques	Relaxation techniques	Relaxation techniques	Relaxation techniques	Relaxation techniques

Fifth phase

Monday	Tuesday	Wednesday	Thursday	Friday	Saturday	Sunday
	Running (at least 30 minutes)			Running (at least 30 minutes)		Swimming
Trigger point massage			Nerve mobilization			
	Strengthening			Strengthening		
Stretching	Stretching	Stretching	Stretching	Stretching	Stretching	Stretching
Relaxation techniques	Relaxation techniques	Relaxation techniques	Relaxation techniques	Relaxation techniques	Relaxation techniques	Relaxation techniques

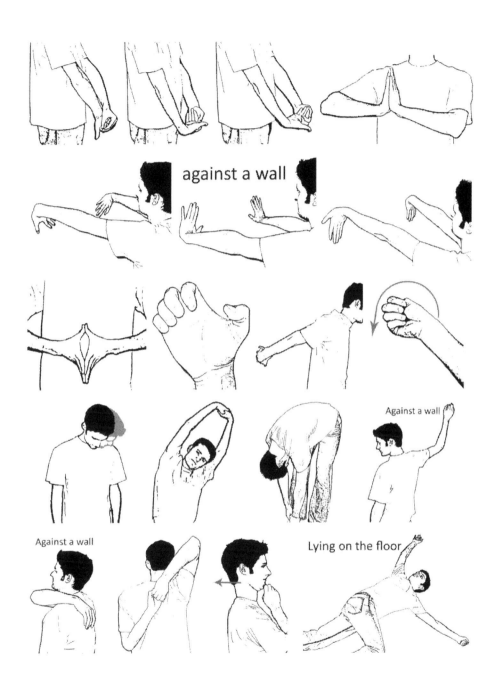

against a wall

Against a wall

Against a wall

Lying on the floor

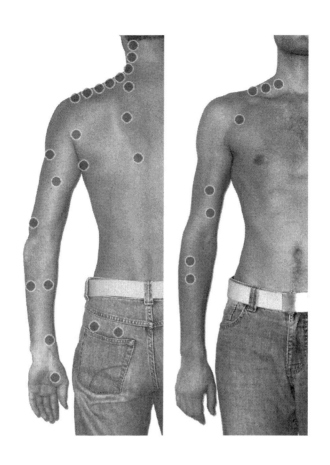

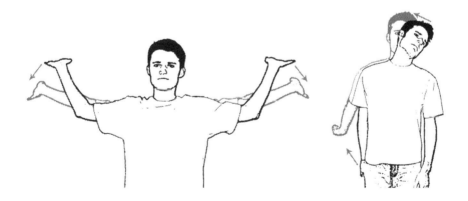

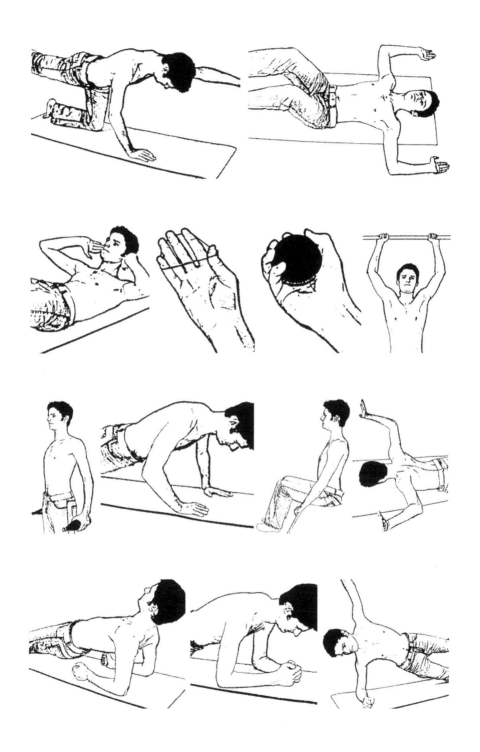

"Normal"	Shortcut	Description
Right-click > Cut	Ctrl + X	Cuts the selected text / object
Right-click > Copy	Ctrl + C	Copies the selected text / object
Right-click > Paste	Ctrl + V	Inserts the selected text / object
Edit > Undo	Ctrl + Z	Undo the last action
Edit > Redo	Ctrl + Y	Reverse an undo command
Multiple keystrokes (arrow keys)	Ctrl + Arrow key	Moves the cursor before / behind a word
Multiple keystrokes (delete / backspace)	Ctrl + Del / Backspace	Deletes a word (Del = behind the mouse cursor, Backspace = before)
Scrolling with the mouse	Page up	Scrolls up one page
Scrolling with the mouse	Page down	Scrolls down one page
Arrow keys or clicking with the mouse	Pos1	Document: Moves the cursor to the beginning of the current line Website: Jumps to the top of the page
Arrow keys or clicking with the mouse	End	Document: Moves the cursor to the end of the current line Website: Jumps to the bottom of the page
Drag the scrollbar with the mouse	Ctrl + Pos1	Moves the cursor to the beginning of a document
Drag the scrollbar with the mouse	Ctrl + End	Moves the cursor to the end of a document
Highlight with the mouse	Ctrl + Shift + Arrow key	Highlights a word
Highlight with the mouse	Shift + Pos1	Highlights everything from the cursor position to the beginning of the current line
Highlight with the mouse	Shift + End	Highlights everything from the cursor position to the end of the current line
Double-click on "My Computer" (this icon is usually only available on the desktop)	Win + E	Opens the Explorer
View > Refresh or - if available - by clicking on a special button in the menu bar	F5	Refreshes the current view (Explorer, Internet Explorer, Firefox etc.)
Left-click on a program in the taskbar	Alt + Tab	Switches between open windows (you can hold Alt and press the Tab key several times)

computer-related
PAIN ?

rsipain.com

rsipain.com rsipain.com rsipain.com rsipain.com rsipain.com rsipain.com rsipain.com rsipain.com rsipain.com rsipain.com rsipain.com rsipain.com rsipain.com rsipain.com rsipain.com rsipain.com

Printed in Great Britain
by Amazon